A SUCCESSFUL NEW YOU

through these simple daily assignments:

Drink lots of water

Bend and stretch

Take a morning walk

Keep track of what you put in your mouth

Watch your servings and portions

Watch your intake of unhealthy fats

Move through the day

SOUNDS SIMPLE? IT IS.

It's like having your own personal trainer,
nutritionist, and physician by your side
every day, and every step of the way
for the rest of your life.

THIN OVER 40

The Simple 12-Week Plan
for Getting Back
the Body You Had . . .
or Building the Body
You've Always Wanted

Gregory L. Jantz, Ph.D.
with Ann McMurray

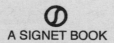

A SIGNET BOOK

SIGNET
Published by New American Library, a division of
Penguin Group (USA) Inc., 375 Hudson Street,
New York, New York 10014, USA
Penguin Group (Canada), 10 Alcorn Avenue, Toronto,
Ontario M4V 3B2, Canada (a division of Pearson Penguin Canada Inc.)
Penguin Books Ltd., 80 Strand, London WC2R 0RL, England
Penguin Ireland, 25 St. Stephen's Green, Dublin 2,
Ireland (a division of Penguin Books Ltd.)
Penguin Group (Australia), 250 Camberwell Road, Camberwell, Victoria 3124,
Australia (a division of Pearson Australia Group Pty. Ltd.)
Penguin Books India Pvt. Ltd., 11 Community Centre, Panchsheel Park,
New Delhi - 110 017, India
Penguin Group (NZ), Cnr Airborne and Rosedale Roads, Albany,
Auckland 1310, New Zealand (a division of Pearson New Zealand Ltd.)
Penguin Books (South Africa) (Pty.) Ltd., 24 Sturdee Avenue,
Rosebank, Johannesburg 2196, South Africa

Penguin Books Ltd., Registered Offices:
80 Strand, London WC2R 0RL, England

First published by Signet, an imprint of New American Library,
a division of Penguin Group (USA) Inc.

First Printing, December 2004
10 9 8 7 6 5 4 3 2 1

PUBLISHER'S NOTE
Every effort as been made to ensure that the information contained in this
book is complete and accurate. However, neither the publisher nor the author
is engaged in rendering professional advice or services to the individual
reader. The ideas, procedures, and suggestions contained in this book are not
intended as a substitute for consulting with your physician. All matters regarding your health require medical supervision. Neither the author nor the
publishers shall be liable or responsible for any loss or damage allegedly
arising from any information or suggestion in this book.

THIN OVER 40

INTRODUCTION

Thin over 40—the holy grail of middle age. Just ask those vainly trying to recapture the body they had (or wanted to have) at twenty. The frustration is tremendous. Many of the weight-loss strategies—fad diets or rigorous, exercise routines—that were successful at age twenty or thirty are no longer as effective. The overriding question becomes, *"Now that I'm over forty, why can't I seem to lose weight?"*

It didn't hit me the day I turned forty; it was a little while after that. Because of a speaking engagement, I needed to get an updated photo of myself. Pretty standard. I'd had the last one done about five years earlier. The photographer came in and took several shots. I didn't give it much thought—until the proofs came back. The earlier picture was clearly of a man in his thirties. The new one was of a man obviously in his forties. I stared at the proofs and thought, *When did this happen?*

The two photos told the story. In five years, I'd increased not just in age, but in size. Frankly, I hadn't paid attention. I was busy with work and family. Even though I counsel people on nutrition, I'd stopped paying as much attention to my own body and weight. It showed. I decided it was time to put into practice the lessons I'd learned from my years of working with those struggling to overcome eating disorders. The result is *Thin over 40*.

As the founder of The Center for Counseling and Health Resources, Inc., I am a certified eating disorder specialist and a nationally certified psychologist. For the past eighteen years at The Center, we have treated nearly seven thousand individuals with weight and food-related issues. I've seen firsthand how these successful strategies help people become *Thin over 40*.

If you're over forty, and think you've lost the "Battle of the Bulge," don't give up! Over the next twelve weeks, through the *Thin over 40 Plan*, you'll:

- Integrate the *5 Success Essentials* to achieving and maintaining *Thin over 40* as a long-term lifestyle change instead of merely a diet or exercise plan for a set amount of weeks.
- Start each day with a motivational reading and interactive assignment.
- Appreciate and enjoy your body through daily moving and stretching.
- Discover what's holding you back so you can move forward.
- Focus each week on a different Key Concept, designed to enhance your *Thin over 40* success.
- Engage daily in the Plan through the Success in Action section.
- Learn the latest health and nutritional information specifically targeted to those over forty.
- Gain an understanding of how you can turn your age from a liability to an asset in your goal to be *Thin over 40*.
- Combat the self-sabotage practiced by so many over forty that dooms long-term success.
- Strategize intentional alternatives to counteract the emotional pull of food, especially sugars and carbohydrates.
- Use the latest research on how to jump start me

tabolism to enhance weight loss through natural, healthy methods.
- Ferret out potential success busters, such as food allergies and sensitivities.

The *Thin over 40* Plan

There are Five Success Essentials to the *Thin over 40* Plan. You may be surprised to see how simple they are. This isn't rocket science but common sense. (No, it isn't rocket science—for some of you it's been a whole lot harder! But it doesn't need to be such a struggle.) Over the next twelve weeks, I'll help you integrate each of these Five Success Essentials into your daily life. They are:

Success Essential #1: Intentional, healthy food and eating choices
Success Essential #2: Increased physical movement
Success Essential #3: Nutritional and hormonal support
Success Essential #4: Restful, curative sleep
Success Essential #5: Proper hydration

Simply put, the Plan will help you eat healthily, move more, utilize the right supplements, get your proper rest, and drink water. This is not the formula for a fad diet but, rather, a lifelong strategy for achieving increased longevity, greater energy, healthy body weight, and freedom from perpetual dieting. It is about enjoying who you are again instead of constantly fretting over your age and your weight.

The *Thin over 40* Plan is about doing, and it's also about understanding. Each week you'll focus on a different Key Concept, designed to enlighten you about your over-forty mind, body, and spirit. Here are the Key Concepts you'll be focusing on each week, as you actively and intentionally replace faulty habits with healthy, proactive lifestyle choices:

Week 1:
Making the Most of You
(Key Concept—Awareness)

We know we need to live and eat healthier, but few of us are aware of how our habits, accumulated up to this point in life, are holding us back from achieving the success we desire. This first week will focus on you—your habits and choices.

WEEK 2:
Making the Most of Your Future
(Key Concept—Longevity)

Diets don't work because they are about restriction and deprivation. The *Thin over 40* Plan is not a diet but a way of life that emphasizes good health and belief in a vibrant future. This vision for your personal future will provide a foundation for continued success.

WEEK 3:
Making the Most of Moving
(Key Concept—Metabolism)

You've got to get your metabolism back on track. As we age, we have a tendency to slow down. It's time to get back into gear and our bodies in motion again with enjoyable, uplifting physical activities, as well as strategic nutrition to assist the body in returning to youthful metabolic levels.

WEEK 4:
Making the Most of Nutrition
(Key Concept—Food and Mood)

What you eat affects how you feel. The latest research proves a definitive link between proper nutrition and a positive, optimistic mind-set. It's time to get your body and mind working together to support your desire to change!

WEEK 5:
Making the Most of Supplements
(Key Concept—Adrenal Health)

Often our over-forty stressful lifestyles take a toll on our adrenal and thyroid systems, contributing to frustrating weight gain. When your adrenal system is stressed or overworked, it automatically causes your thyroid to "turn down" your metabolic rate to calm your system. A reduced metabolism can mean increased weight.

WEEK 6:
Making the Most of Your Brain
(Key Concept—Brain Power)

Four powerful brain chemicals—GABA, endorphins, dopamine, and serotonin—regulate how you respond to pleasure, stress, and pain. For many, food has become a way to deal with those situations instead. By putting your neurotransmitters back in charge, food loses its draw.

WEEK 7:
Making the Most of Rest
(Key Concept—Rest)

For many of us, the difficulties and stresses of life over forty sap our energy. We're tired and depressed, and it seems too hard to make needed changes. Though there are many reasons for fatigue, sometimes it's as simple as not getting the rest we need each day. There's tremendous power in a good night's sleep.

WEEK 8:
Making the Most of "The Change"
(Key Concept—Hormones)

This week is devoted to the physiological effects of both menopause and the male version, adropause. When hormone levels drop, especially after age forty, your body reacts significantly! These changes must be factored into the *Thin over 40* lifestyle.

WEEK 9:
Making the Most of Balance
(Key Concept—Balance)

Sometimes a craving is just a craving, but sometimes impulsive eating is caused by hidden food allergies or food sensitivities that sabotage our best intentions. By cutting down on the number and severity of cravings, you'll feel better, think clearer, and weigh less.

WEEK 10:
Making the Most of Relationships
(Key Concept—Relationships)

Many of those over forty have developed a convenient yet unhealthy relationship with food. It provides comfort, stress relief, affirmation, a break from boredom. Under the *Thin over 40* Plan, food returns to being nutrition, leaving plenty of room for healthy, positive relationships with the important *people* in your life.

WEEK 11:
Making the Most of Forgiveness
(Key Concept—Forgiveness)

Thin over 40 is a not a diet but a lifestyle. You will experience times of forward momentum and you will backslide a time or two. This is normal, yet many people respond to a step backward by stopping altogether. Don't forget that two steps forward and one step back is still progress. Each step backward can provide valuable lessons for navigating future roadblocks.

WEEK 12:
Making the Most of Life
(Key Concept—Success)

Now that you've embarked on a lifelong commitment to your health and future, it's important to take time to remember and appreciate your success. This celebration of your progress will help motivate you to continue to reinforce your areas of success and strengthen those areas that may still persist as challenges.

Twelve weeks, or three months. That's the length of time I'm asking for. Here's what else I'm asking for:

- *Start on a Monday.* Begin the *Thin over 40* Plan on a Monday, as weekends can be a difficult time to begin changing habits.
- *Stick with it.* If you find you've gone off the Plan, get back on it and start again.
- *Be the Plan.* Don't just read about it, actually do it. Don't shortchange yourself by shortchanging the Plan.
- *Trust me.* Trust me until you can trust yourself.
- *Don't put it off.* Start right now, not next month or some unnamed date in the future, because your health and your tomorrow are worth it.
- *Expect success.* Your attitude will be the driving

factor in so many of the positive changes you'll be making. The smaller your expectations, the smaller your success. The greater your optimism, the greater your ability to implement these life-enhancing actions.

- *Give it one more shot.* I know that many of you have tried myriad other methods and even now you're listening to that "nothing's worked" voice in your mind. Don't listen. I've reviewed over seventy-five books and read reams of research. The elements of *Thin over 40* are effective. I've seen it in others and am living it myself today. This will work!

Over the next twelve weeks, you're going to start each morning with this book. It will motivate you, keep you on track, and give you direction. For that reason, don't put off reading! Do it the first thing when you wake up in the morning and give yourself adequate time to go over each day's Thin Thought, Setting the Day for Success, Success in Action and other information provided. You're setting the tone for each day to become *Thin over 40*.

Please remember that the *Thin over 40* Plan is not a lose-weight-quick-only-to-gain-it-back-and-moresystem. Will you lose weight? Yes. But for many of you, the amount of weight you need to lose in order to achieve a healthy goal will take longer than the twelve weeks. And that's perfectly fine. It is what you are learning, doing, and understanding *during* the twelve weeks that will set you on a course for success to lose that weight—no matter how much it is. Haven't we all had enough of those get-thin-quick diets that work for a brief moment in time but then return us to our previous weight, and more?

Self-imposed restrictive diets that produce quick and dramatic results have a tendency to boomerang with a subsequent weight gain. The best results are achieved through a long-term, realistic drop of one to two pounds per week. The goal of this plan is not to help you take off twenty pounds in May so you'll be ready for summer, or drop ten pounds before your daughter's wedding or upcoming high-school reunion. It's not a panic, event-driven diet. Rather, it's a plan to redirect you toward nurturing your body through healthy living and renewing your mind through a positive self-image.

The key person involved in the Plan is not me, it's you. You are the one to take the information and concepts presented and put them into practice for yourself. For this reason, there is not a regimented daily list of what to eat and how much. Rather, over the course of the next twelve weeks, you'll gain insight into what you eat and why. Then you can decide for yourself how you want to implement the necessary changes in your everyday life. It is not up to me to tell you to eat a broccoli salad every Wednesday for lunch. It is up to me to warn you of the dangers of consuming too high a percentage of unhealthy fat calories each day. Granted, I have daily assignments for you, but they're designed to allow you to explore your own reasons for eating and to develop personal solutions tailored to your life.

Why not just tell you what to eat every day? Because I want you to develop the ability over the next twelve weeks to create each day's menu for yourself, using the information and insights provided. In this way, even when you put the book down, you'll have gained the skills to continue on your own. That is the goal—for you to keep with this Plan for life! I recently read a study that said women stay on a diet an average of only four weeks, and men only six weeks—with the specific goal of losing weight. The diets are generally restrictive in nature and they do lose weight. However, they immediately gain the weight back as soon as they go off the diet. This is not beneficial. This is not the *Thin over 40* way. Allow yourself the freedom to try different foods, become more informed about what you eat and why, and integrate these choices—your choices—over the next twelve weeks.

Throughout the book you're going to receive a great deal of information, inspiration, and motivation. These will be provided in small, daily amounts instead of in chapter form, as many books use. This is very intentional: It's not just about giving you the information, it's also about developing habits, integrating changes, and learning to take daily baby steps toward a *Thin over 40* life. Read your daily section; take in the information and the insights and allow them to work their way down into your core convictions. It's more than about information; it's about understanding. It's also about time—give yourself the time to practice these concepts in your own life. Be patient. Be diligent. Be optimistic!

The first thing I want you to do is purchase a journal. Choose any kind you like, from a plain spiral-bound version to a fancy, fabric-covered book. The outside isn't what's important. I want you to use this journal over the next twelve weeks. You're going to be writing down how you feel about yourself, your life, your body, your future. This is really a case of you helping yourself succeed.

Let's face it, one of the advantages of being over forty is the maturity we've gained along the way, which allows us to make intentional, positive changes. We've learned how to work hard toward a goal. We've learned how to say no to some things in order to say yes to others. We've experienced success and gratification in many aspects of our lives and careers. Now it's time to take all of that knowledge, experience, and maturity, and put them to work on the one thing you've probably neglected in attaining the others—your body and your health.

It's time. Let's get started!

WEEK 1
MAKING THE MOST OF YOU

WEEK 1 ❧ DAY 1

Today's Thin Thought: Today is the first day of the rest of your life.

Good morning! Congratulations on your decision to integrate the *Thin over 40* Plan into your life! Take a moment to say out loud today's Thin Thought. Personalize it. Internalize it. Live it—love it— embrace it! Whatever you've tried in the past, whatever you have or haven't done, don't let that stop you. Commit to today, for the sake of today. Your goal is to look to the future, not be encumbered by the past.

During the next twelve weeks, you'll be taking positive steps to increase your energy, reduce unwanted pounds, and improve your vitality and longevity—through a life-enhancing plan instead of the bondage of restrictive dieting. The goal is to help you intentionally undergo a realistic, healthful, long-term lifestyle transformation. Now that you're over forty, it's time to readjust how you think about yourself and how you fuel your body. It's time to reexamine the ways you deal with food. It's time to fall in love with your body again (or for the first time) and appreciate how a healthy lifestyle can benefit you from this day forward, no matter your age.

1

SETTING THE DAY FOR SUCCESS

Let's go over the Five Success Essentials you'll be working on over the next twelve weeks:

Success Essential #1: Intentional, healthy food and eating choices
Success Essential #2: Increased physical movement
Success Essential #3: Nutritional and hormonal support
Success Essential #4: Restful, curative sleep
Success Essential #5: Proper hydration

We'll be adding on to each of these, but as a start, I want you to begin a couple right away.

Your daily assignments:
- **Drink lots of water.**
- **Bend, stretch, and move upon waking.**
- **Walk in the morning for at least fifteen minutes.**

And I do mean right away! Go get yourself a large glass of water, if you don't have one already. (I'll wait for you to get back.)

From now on, I want you to keep water with you at all times. It is important for you to drink at least two quarts of water each day. Yes, half a gallon of water each and every day! If that seems like more than you could possibly drink, think about it this way: How many of you have gone to 7-Eleven for a Big Gulp of pop? Big Gulps are thirty-two ounces—one quart—and half of your water consumption. Super Big Gulps are even larger at forty-four ounces. Two quarts seems like a lot because it's water and you're not used to it. (I live in Seattle with some of the sweetest, best-tasting tap water in the country. You may not be so fortunate. You may want to choose bottled water if you live in a part of the country that has, frankly, lousy-tasting tap water. If you've got older plumbing, you should also drink bottled water to avoid consuming some of the heavy metals that can leech into tap water through old systems. You don't have to choose pricey, designer water. Most grocery stores have large, inexpensive gallon jugs of water.)

If it still seems daunting, try this—drink one cup, or eight ounces, of water upon rising each morning. Keep a cup of water on your nightstand so you can drink it immediately upon waking. Drink another cup before each meal. Violà! You'll have had half your water, leaving you just another four cups to drink during the day. Many people keep a quart-sized water bottle alongside them during the day, sipping periodically. At first, it may seem strange, but you'll quickly become used to it as just a part of your day. Relax, it's not as hard as you think!

What about drinking other liquids during the day, like coffee, tea, alcohol or soft drinks? Because these drinks often have a diuretic effect (cause you to lose water), you'll need to drink twice as much extra water. In other words, if you drink a twelve-ounce soda, you'll need to consume an extra twenty-four ounces, or three cups, of water. If it's not worth it to you, then try foregoing these beverages. You may be surprised to realize that once you stop consuming the other beverages and drink primarily water, you'll actually crave them less as your body is properly hydrated.

Why so much water? We're made up mostly of water. Water is our bodies' lubricant. When we don't get enough, the body doesn't function well. We experience fatigue. Our metabolism slows down. We feel lethargic and crabby. We end up eating something to make us feel better, misinterpreting thirst for hunger.

Okay, you've got your water. Here's the other thing you need to do each day in the morning. I want you to get up out of bed and stretch. Just do a couple minutes of moving, bending, and stretching your body, while taking deep breaths. You're basically telling your body it's time to wake up and get in gear. For many of us over forty, we've forgotten what our bodies *feel* like when we move and stretch. Remember, your body is not your enemy. Part of this stretching is to reacquaint you with your body, to regain an appreciation so you'll be motivated to continue with these and other healthy choices. Stretch your arms, back, legs. Your torso. Allow your muscles and joints to achieve gentle full extension, while increasing blood flow to all parts of your body. This will help you wake up and get set for the day.

For every single one of you who is able, I want you to get out every morning—yes, every morning, rain or shine—and take at least a fifteen-minute walk. *But I can't walk that long,* you may say. Well, try fifteen minutes. If you can't go that long, go as long as you can. The goal over the next twelve weeks is for you to gradually increase your physical activity and walking is a wonderful way to get outside and move! Breathe deeply, taking measured full-lung breaths.

Commit to doing this each day in the morning. If you want to take an additional walk or exercise in the afternoon or evening, that's great! You still need to get up and move and get out and walk each morning. Moving in the morning triggers an increase in metabolism that lasts into the day. This movement also improves your mood through the release of endorphins, your body's natural opiates.

Right now, drink another cup of water and do

your stretching. Then put on a comfortable pair of shoes and get out into your neighborhood. Enjoy fifteen minutes of time that's just for you. Use a radio headset or portable CD player if you like. Walk as briskly as you can, knowing you'll be able to increase the speed and the duration over the next several weeks. Above all, don't concern yourself with what you can't do; concentrate instead on taking advantage of what you can. When you get back from your walk, get out your journal and take a few minutes to complete the Success in Action section.

SUCCESS IN ACTION

In your journal, answer the following questions. Be honest and open with your answers.

- List three reasons why you want to be *Thin over 40*.
- Envision how a typical day will be better with your new *Thin over 40* lifestyle.
- Name three obstacles you expect and are committed to overcome in your goal to be *Thin over 40*.
- Don't be limited to these questions. Allow yourself to document whatever you feel important. It's your journal. It's your life.

Today, focus on keeping your water with you and becoming aware of how you feel at various parts of the day. Remember, the Key Concept is Awareness.

WEEK 1 🦋 DAY 2

Today's Thin Thought: You are what you eat.

Your daily assignments:
- **Drink lots of water.**
- **Bend, stretch, and move upon waking.**

- **Walk in the morning for at least fifteen minutes.**
- **Keep track of what you put in your mouth.**

Good morning! Welcome to Day 2! Had your water yet? How did your stretching go? If you haven't had your water or moved your body to welcome today, put down the book and do both. A routine doesn't happen by thinking about it; it happens by doing. So make sure you do it every day. It's not that much to ask.

SETTING THE DAY FOR SUCCESS

Look again at today's Thin Thought and make it your own—*I am what I eat.* While we know the truth of that statement, we often don't pay attention to what, and how much, we actually do eat. By forty and beyond, much of our eating habits are just that—habits. We eat without thinking. From the foods we choose, to the times and places we eat, it's time to bring some awareness into our desire to be *Thin over 40.*

From now on, each day, I want you to write down what you eat. That way, you'll know. Use your journal and draw yourself a grid with these headings, one for today and each day this week:

Date	Time	What Eaten	Location	Estimated Calories

You can also keep track of cups of water you're drinking by making a hash mark for each cup on the page. Your goal is simply to track what you eat. That means *everything*. If it's not water, it's food. (I realize tea, black coffee, and diet drinks don't have any calories, but I want you to track how much you're drinking so you can consume twice the amount of water to compensate.) Again, I want you to track every bit of food you put in your mouth—meals, snacks, munching, nibbling, everything. Take the journal with you wherever you go throughout this week. (Don't be self-conscious about it. Other people don't know what it's for.)

Please note: I'm not asking you to change what you're eating at this point. Rather, I want you to realize how much you're eating and how often during the day you eat. Remember, this week's Key Concept is Awareness.

In order to estimate calories, look at the packaging for nutritional information. Do the best you can, estimating when specifics aren't present. This isn't scientific research; it's an exercise in self-discovery. Before you can alter entrenched patterns, you need to know and understand what they are. You also need to be aware of any "danger zones" to your eating—in other words, times or places that present a particular challenge to you. By keeping track, these patterns will become evident. If you've never tracked calories like this before, prepare to be surprised. Calories add up quickly. Even if the amount seems "too big," write it down anyway. This will help you become more aware of the actual impact of your favorite foods.

Again, this is to build awareness, not *obsession*. Believe me when I tell you that twenty years of work with eating disorders has allowed me to see the damage done to lives through an obsession with food, weight, and body image. The *Thin over 40* Plan is not designed to train you to obsess about these things. All we want to do is recognize general patterns, which will give you insight into your own behaviors. As you gain knowledge and understanding, you can disconnect from these behaviors to reintegrate new, healthier ones. Once these new behaviors are fully integrated, you can discontinue the daily tracking because eating healthy will become part of who you are, not merely what you do. I do want you to continue to track your food during the full twelve weeks of *Thin over 40*.

As a bonus this week, write down any time you *wanted* to eat something but decided it wasn't worth it because you'd have to write it down. Realize that without the simple constraint of the journal, you probably would have eaten it. All of these calories, eaten either in large meals or in small, constant bites during the day, add up and add weight.

SUCCESS IN ACTION

Make sure you take the time to prepare your food log. For those of you who are cringing at the thought of keeping track of everything you eat, remember: The only person who needs to see this is you. The only person you are accountable to is you. Ask yourself what harm you think will come of tracking what you eat. Write down the biggest reason you don't want to track your food consumption. Now, examine what other reasons might be lurking behind that reason you've put down. Perhaps you think it will be too time-consuming. Is the real reason because you don't want to acknowledge the amounts and types of food you eat each day? Perhaps you think it won't really matter and you can do the Plan without it. Is the real reason because you don't want to be presented with the truth of your eating habits and what they're doing to your health? Is the real reason because you want to remain in control of what, when, and how you eat? If that's the case, then why did you pick up this book? *Talk your way through your objections and stick with the Plan!*

WEEK 1 🦋 DAY 3

Today's Thin Thought: When finding answers, half the battle is knowing the question.

Your daily assignments:
- Drink lots of water.
- Bend, stretch, and move upon waking.
- Walk in the morning for at least fifteen minutes.
- Keep track of what you put in your mouth.

Your weekly assignment:
- Weigh yourself.

SETTING THE DAY FOR SUCCESS

Good morning to you and welcome to Day 3! You are working this week to increase your awareness of when you eat, how much you eat, and where you eat. Today, let's focus on what you eat or, more specific, what you have to eat at home. Our kitchens are where we "relax" where food is concerned. Each of us has staples—milk, flour, rice, canned goods, etc. In that, we'll be pretty similar. Go to anyone's kitchen and you'll see like items. But keep digging through freezers and cabinets, and you'll find the special comfort foods that all of us make sure to keep handy. These are generally the ice cream, cookies, baked goods, chips, processed desserts, and snack items. In and of themselves, these foods are not wrong or bad. In fact, many are great! So great, that we tend to choose them over other foods too much of the time.

At some point today, go through your kitchen, including your refrigerator, freezer, and cabinets. Record all of the dessert and snack items you find in the following way:

- Name of the item
- Number of servings per package
- Amount of calories in each serving
- Number of servings times calories per serving
- Amount of fat calories in each serving
- Number of servings times fat calories per serving
- Amount of sodium in each serving
- Number of servings times sodium per serving
- Number of grams of carbohydrates in each serving
- Number of servings times carbohydrates per serving

After you've gone through and tallied your package totals, calculate a grand total for all of that comfort food. My guess is that it will be in the thousands of calories. Take the grand total and divide by 3,500—the amount of calories needed to make a pound. All of those items together represent a good portion of the excess weight you want to shed!

After you've done this, you can put it all back where you found it. The point of this exercise is not to insist you can't have your favorite chocolate-chip cookies. It's about Awareness. We'll talk more about this as we continue on through the following weeks. For now, it's enough for you to become aware of the caloric impact of your comfort foods.

SUCCESS IN ACTION

I want you to go into your bathroom and weigh yourself. You're going to be weighing yourself every week on the third day of each week so it will be consistent. Because weight fluctuates daily, I don't want you to live or die by the scale.

If you haven't been drinking enough water in the past, your body is used to being dehydrated as a constant condition. In order to adjust, your body has developed a strategy of water retention. In other words, it retains the fluid you drink in your tissues because you're not drinking enough for it to let go. As you rehydrate yourself, your body will take a few days to figure out this isn't just a fluke and you're actually going to start a habit of providing it the water it needs. At first, you'll feel bloated because your tissues are being saturated with water. You'll also go to the bathroom frequently because of the increased consumption. Don't be concerned! Your body will adjust. By drinking more water, you'll actually retain less water and your kidneys will adjust so you won't feel like you need to go to the bathroom every two minutes. Initially, however, your weight may increase because of the water retention. This is a temporary condition—don't panic!

Besides, the scale is not a measure of your worth as a person. Rather, it's a measurement tool for your current body weight. Working for almost twenty years helping those with eating disorders, I am not a fan of daily weighing. I've seen far too many people who are controlled—to the point of endangering their health—by what the scales read.

Weigh yourself today and write it down. You will want to determine how much weight loss is a healthy, realistic amount for you. Using the body mass index, find a healthy weight goal for yourself.

You can calculate your own BMI by taking your weight in pounds multiplied by 703 and divide by your height in inches, squared. Let's try an example: If you are 5 feet 4 inches tall and weigh 150 lbs, your BMI would be 25.74. That's 150 (your weight in pounds) x 703 divided by 64 squared (your height in inches) or 4096. (I live in Seattle, the home of Bill Gates and Microsoft so I am naturally enamored with the Internet. If you would like to calculate your BMI online, you can go to www.consumer.gov/weightloss/bmi/htm. This helpful site has an automatic BMI calculation feature. Put in your height and weight to obtain your current BMI. You can also put in your goal weight and determine what BMI that represents.) A healthy BMI is between 19 and 25. A person is considered obese at a BMI of 30 while a range of 26 to 29 is considered moderately over-weight. Determine your current BMI and then calculate what your weight would need to be to move you into a more healthy range, subtracting the second from the first. This is the amount of excess weight you'll want to use as a goal to lose. For some of you, losing this amount of weight in twelve weeks will be realistic. For some of you, it will not. The *Thin over 40* Plan is not a guarantee to get down to your goal weight in twelve weeks. It's meant to set you upon a path of healthy choices that will *include* weight loss, as a natural consequence of your decisions. Studies show that slow, consistent weight loss produces greater success for keeping the weight off. By shedding excess weight slowly, through lifestyle changes instead of self-imposed starvation, you'll be solidifying these positive habits for the rest of your life.

WEEK 1 🦋 DAY 4

Today's Thin Thought: Knowledge is power.

It's time for Day 4 of *Thin over 40*! Drink and stretch. Drink and stretch. Greet the day head-on. Try turning your body from side to side as you stretch. Extend the muscles from the tips of your fingers to the ends of your toes, and all parts in between. Learn how your body feels when it moves. Learn your body. Love your body. It's not your enemy.

Your daily assignments:
- **Drink lots of water.**
- **Bend, stretch, and move upon waking.**
- **Walk in the morning for at least fifteen minutes.**
- **Keep track of what you put in your mouth.**
- **Watch your servings.**

SETTING THE DAY FOR SUCCESS

You've gone through your kitchen and realized how many calories are represented in your comfort foods. There is a second part to this exercise that I'd like you to become more aware of today. It's the concept of portions or servings. Today I'd like you to begin tracking how many servings you eat at a sitting. For example, do you have three servings of mashed potatoes with your roast at dinner? Is your afternoon snack a serving and a half of milk and two servings (or three) of cookies? In the morning, are you eating two servings of cereal?

It is important to your awareness to actually measure your portions. Eat as normal, taking the quantity you usually take. For example, get out your cereal bowl and pour the amount that is normal for you. But then I want you to get out a measuring cup and find out how much that actually is. You could find that instead of your bowl of cereal being the 160 calories it says on the box, it actually represents 2 servings, or 320 calories, or more. Add a glass of juice, some toast or bagel with butter and jam, and your breakfast could wind up being upward of 800 calories.

Now, as you continue with your food log, you'll be better able to track the actual number of servings and calories your normal meals represent. Add a column, anywhere you can, that tracks servings eaten. Even if the numbers seem high to you, don't be discouraged. Focus on the knowledge and insight this exercise is providing you! Knowledge is power!

SUCCESS IN ACTION

Your assignment for today is to obtain a copy of the federal government's Food Guide Pyramid. (Yes, it's changing in 2005, but it is still good for you to use as a base for food choice decisions. From what I've read, the changes in 2005 will only put it more in line with the *Thin over 40* Plan!) The Food Guide Pyramid gives recommended servings of each of the five food groups (vegetable group; bread, cereal, rice, and pasta group; fruit group; milk, yogurt, and cheese group; meat, poultry, fish, dry beans, eggs, and nuts group; and fats, oils, and sweets group). It provides an excellent guideline for you to use as you work toward finding the combination that's right for you.

If you have access to the Internet, either at home, at work, or through your public library, you can obtain a copy by going to www.pueblo.gsa.gov/cic_text/food/food-pyramid/main.htm. You will be able to print out a multipage report outlining the Food Guide Pyramid and healthy eating tips. Specific to today, it also contains invaluable information on what constitutes a serving of various common foods, and what percentage of fats, sodium, and sugars make up what you've eaten. This is wonderful information! Don't put off getting your copy today. Keep it handy and available for future planning. (For an idea of what the new 2005 Food Guide Pyramid might look like, you can go to www.healthyliving.org/newsletter/ 2003/01newpyramid.html. It separates out "good" fats from "bad" fats.) The new Food Pyramid coming out in 2005 will emphasize "good" fats, whole grains and cereals. Go to any Internet search engine and type in "New Food Pyramid" to see articles and graphics of what the new pyramid will look like.

In your journal, I want you to write down three of your favorite "healthy" foods, why you like them, and their benefits. Then write down three of your favorite "unhealthy" foods, why you like them, and their negative health consequences. Try to choose not only full dishes but also foods that could be considered "snacks." During the course of the next twelve weeks, substitute one of your favorite healthy foods for one recurring unhealthy choice. Your goal is to turn that healthy food into a regular in your diet and switch that unhealthy choice from regular to occasional.

It's time to modify your food log by expanding from tracking calories alone to tracking calories, fats, carbohydrates, proteins, and sodium. The calories in everything you eat will come from fats, carbohydrates, or proteins. Why track sodium? Many manufacturers pump up the amount of sodium in low-fat, lite foods to enhance the taste. Too much sodium can lead to high blood pressure and water retention.

Begin today to keep a daily food log in your journal. Set it up this way (you will probably need to turn the page, so you are writing at its widest part):

Date	Time	What Eaten	Where	Calories	Carbs/Protein/Fats (grams)	Sodium (mg)

Don't worry You won't need to do this forever, just until you build a realistic awareness of the nutritional consequences of your food choices. Continue to keep track and we'll talk more about the implications next week and why it's important to track grams of carbohydrates, proteins, and fats. For now, whenever possible, just note that information off the labels of the foods you eat. (If you have a question about a product without a label, please see the Resource List for information on Dr. Phil McGraw's *The Ultimate Weight Solution Food Guide*. Chances are, you'll be able to find an item close enough to yours to estimate fairly accurately.)

WEEK 1   🦋   DAY 5

Today's Thin Thought: Eternal vigilance is the price of freedom.

Your daily assignments:
- **Drink lots of water.**
- **Bend, stretch, and move upon waking.**
- **Walk in the morning for at least fifteen minutes.**
- **Keep track of what you put in your mouth.**
- **Watch your servings.**

Thank you for allowing me to paraphrase Thomas Jefferson for today's Thin Thought. It illustrates that freedom from excess weight and poor food habits comes through consistent awareness and action. This week, you've gone through your kitchen and are becoming more aware of the food you surround yourself with and the impact it has on your weight and health. We want to extend that good work to other areas.

.

SETTING THE DAY FOR SUCCESS

Today I want you to go through your work space and personal vehicles. If you work from home, go through the areas you use as a home office. What you are looking for are those stashes of food that many of us keep in our workplaces and cars. If you look in the drawers of your coworkers, you'll probably find candy or snacks hidden away, just in case. Many times, we think snacking at work doesn't fall under the category of "eating" because it isn't a full meal or we eat those snacks a little bit at a time, over an extended period of time. We have come to consider those calories not to "count" during our day. A cookie here. A candy bar there. Half a bag of chips. A doughnut during break. Because we're distracted when we eat them, we simply forget or fail to notice them in the grand scheme of eating. Compounding matters is the reality that these foods are often the least healthy, with lots of fats, sugars, and sodium. They taste great, get us through the morning and/ or afternoon—and are responsible for extra pounds around our waists and hips.

Workplace eating or vehicle eating is often "hidden" eating. These areas are natural "danger zones" for many of us, where we eat types of foods and amounts we wouldn't particularly care to own up to. It's time to defuse these places by making them no-snack zones.

For now, I'd like you to clear out all of your stashes. Gather them up, put them in a bag. (Hang on to them because you'll be using them later in the Success in Action section for today.) Now, focus on your quart of water, kept on your desk. Every time you feel the need to reach for those chips, that pastry or candy bar, take a sip of water. When you're genuinely hungry, get up and have a full, healthy meal. Enjoy a cookie as dessert afterward—but then don't eat again until dinner in the evening.

Some of you may require a small snack in the afternoon to maintain your glucose-to-insulin ratio. If that is the case, make sure your snack is small and healthy. Try a fruit-and-grain bar, a piece of fruit, or some veggies. Remember, this is a snack and should not have the calories of a full meal.

SUCCESS IN ACTION

After you have gathered up all of the stashes (from wherever you keep them, not just the locations mentioned here; if it's your stash, it still counts!), write them down and add up the calories they represent. In your journal, estimate how many calories each day you'll save by removing these snack items. Since most of the snacking is almost subconscious, you're not going to be missing all that much. By substituting a sip of water instead of that snack, you'll increase your water intake and attain a sense of fullness with something that's good for you!

WEEK 1 🦋 DAY 6

Today's Thin Thought: Success is its own reward.

Your daily assignments:
- **Drink lots of water.**

- Bend, stretch, and move upon waking.
- Walk in the morning for at least fifteen minutes.
- Keep track of what you put in your mouth.
- Watch your servings.

If you began the *Thin over 40* Plan on Monday, Day 6 is a Saturday. For many of you, this constitutes the weekend, a time to take a break from your workplace. No clock to punch. You can just sit back and relax. Well, not quite. You still need to get up, drink your water, and do your stretching. When you get out and walk today, take a family member with you. See if you can go a little bit longer.

SETTING THE DAY FOR SUCCESS

Yes, the weekend can be a wonderful time to relax and refresh. For too many of us, however, relaxing means sitting in our easy chair with the television on, munching nonstop for hours, while sipping our favorite relaxing beverage of choice. It's time for us to rethink the concept of relaxation and disconnect it from only eating and drinking. Today, intentionally choose a different way of unwinding from the week. It might be to get out of the house with family and engage in an enjoyable group activity. It might be tackling that one home project you've put off, knowing how great it will feel when it's checked off your list! It might be to get outside and work in the yard. Or go into the city and view an art exhibit. Whatever it is, find something that engages your mind and involves some amount of physical movement. Bring your water with you and, whenever possible, include a family member or friend.

During today and tomorrow, intentionally choose to save your easy-chair experience for the end of the day. If there's a special television show or sporting event, listen to it on the radio as you work at another task, or record it to be viewed in the evening. Make sure to contain your eating to breakfast, lunch, and dinner. And when you do sit down to eat, relax and enjoy your meal. Take time to catch up with other family members or a good book. Continue to be aware of how much you eat.

SUCCESS IN ACTION

Spend some extra time writing in your journal today. Reflect on what you've learned this week about your eating habits, how much you eat, what your comfort foods are. Recommit to your goal to be *Thin over 40*. Write yourself a promise to keep with it and why. Tell yourself that your life, your health, and your peace of mind are worth the effort!

WEEK 1   🦋   DAY 7

Today's Thin Thought: The best offense is a good defense.

Your daily assignments:
- **Drink lots of water.**
- **Bend, stretch, and move upon waking.**
- **Walk in the morning for at least fifteen minutes.**
- **Keep track of what you put in your mouth.**
- **Watch your servings.**

Weekly Assginment:
- **Go grocery shopping for next week.**

SETTING THE DAY FOR SUCCESS

Congratulations on your first week of *Thin over 40*! I am hopeful that, by today, you're gaining an appreciation for the benefits of being well hydrated and the joy of moving and stretching your body. Continue to do this every morning so you'll develop a lifelong habit. After all, this is no different than brushing your teeth or showering in the morning or doing any number of daily personal hygiene tasks. As we age, these become even more important. They are ways to acknowledge and appreciate our bodies for how far they have taken us, as well as a deposit on their ability to take us even farther. We want to stay healthy and active!

I also hope you are coming to terms with tracking your food consumption and serving amounts. The Key Concept for this week has been Awareness. You have been engaged in activities to help you focus on becoming more aware of your habits and eating patterns. As we look to shift some of those patterns, you want to be proactive in planning for next week. During this week, you've become more aware of what foods and snack items are in your kitchen, at work, and in your car. Today is a perfect day to sit down and make out a grocery list for next week. Record your grocery list in your journal so you can keep track of how it changes during the next twelve weeks. Remember to take your time to think about what foods you want to surround you and nourish you for this upcoming week.

I'm not advocating filling your cart with nothing but carrot sticks and rice cakes. Rather, as you make your list, think of a couple of ways you can use more fruits and vegetables in your dishes this week. Give yourself enough time to shop to be able to really look at the nutritional information on the foods you are considering. Observe the number of servings, and the calories, fats, sugars, and sodium amounts each serving represents. Look for healthier alternatives. Many grocery stores group similar products, so you'll be able to compare the labels from one product to the next. Look for labels at face value, however. Remember to turn that package over or turn that can around and really look at the nutrition label and compare. Instead of your regular sandwich bread, try a whole-grain alternative. Instead of a can of creamed soup, try a broth soup with lower saturated fat. Why not pick up a bag of pretzels instead of potato chips? In response to consumer demand, manufacturers are beginning to provide healthier alternatives to common foods. Learn what's available in your favorite grocery store. Be on the lookout for complimentary recipes often provided in the produce section. Try out a new fruit or vegetable. Try types of foods you haven't eaten before.

Most of all, give yourself time. Grant yourself permission to do this. Too often we become creatures of habit even when it comes to what aisles we go down in the grocery store. Today, go down every aisle and see what's there. Use your list and make choices about what foods you are going to have available to you for breakfast, lunch, and dinner. This doesn't need to turn into a battle zone, a war between what you know you want to eat and what you think you should eat. Talk to yourself about the positive reasons for making healthier choices.

SUCCESS IN ACTION

Before you head off to the grocery store today, make sure to eat a full meal. When you're hungry and you go food shopping, who knows what could end up in that cart! I'm not expecting you to completely change all of your eating habits within this first week but I do want you to begin the process of evaluating what goes into that cart. If you want to put in a half gallon of your favorite ice cream, fine. If you want a package of cookies, that's okay. But the contents of your cart should not be primarily processed foods, desserts, salty snacks, or prepackaged baked goods.

To help you determine how much of what to put in your cart, get out your Food Guide Pyramid and take it with you to the store. If what you're buying is what you're going to be eating this week, look at the serving suggestions for each group and allow your cart to more closely mirror the Pyramid than before. Remember that you are looking to provide balance to what you eat, including carbohydrates, proteins, and fats from a variety of nutrient-rich foods. Write down your grocery list in your journal and then note anything you pick up that isn't on the list. (As a bonus, write down anything you *wanted* to pick up but didn't because you'd have to write it down.)

HERO OF THE WEEK

Each week we'll be focusing on a Hero of the Week. This is a person who has incorporated the aspects of the Plan into his or her life. Their stories are meant to encourage you, motivate you, and give you a boost to keep going. These are everyday people, just like you, who are living *Thin over 40*.

Before we get into the stories of other people, this first week the big story is You! You've kept with the Plan for a full week. You haven't given up. You haven't put the book away. You're still reading. You're still working on your health and becoming *Thin over 40*.

You're the Hero of the Week and you're my hero! Keep it up!

WEEK 2
MAKING THE MOST OF YOUR FUTURE

WEEK 2 🦋 DAY 1

Today's Thin Thought: Positive changes enhance your life.

Welcome to Week 2 of *Thin over 40*! I applaud your continued commitment to achieve a healthy, vibrant, mature lifestyle. This week, you will continue to do the following things:

- **Drink lots of water.** Keep working toward two quarts per day.
- **Bend, stretch, and move upon waking.** Wake up each morning and spend several minutes stretching and moving your body as you physically prepare for the day.
- **Walk in the morning for at least fifteen minutes.** If you are able to do more than that, great! Whenever possible, get outside and walk. If it's December and there's a foot of snow on the ground, you'll have to be more creative. Try going to a local shopping center or indoor mall. Many open up early to allow people to walk inside before the stores open. If there is no shopping center or mall near where you live, consider joining a health club and using a treadmill whenever it's too cold or stormy to be outside, or march, jog, or dance around at home to a 20-

minute exercise video—there is a great variety to choose from. And on every possible day you can, get outside, take advantage, and enjoy it!

- **Keep track of what you put in your mouth.** Build an awareness of your unconscious habits where food is concerned.
- **Watch your servings.** Realize it is possible to live on less.

SETTING THE DAY FOR SUCCESS

The Key Concept for this week is *Longevity*. Most of us want to live a good, long life, full of vitality even as we age. We want to experience health, well into our senior years. Have you ever seen pictures or read interviews with people who have lived to very old age? Occasionally, it will be a person who has "beaten the odds" by living a long life even while engaging in unhealthy habits such as smoking, drinking, or improper eating. That is very rare, however. Most of us recognize that in order to enhance our longevity, we need to make certain lifestyle choices. These choices inevitably involve change. As adults, it can be difficult to change. Even though you're over forty sometimes it's good to go back and review fundamentals learned as children. Let's reenergize and revitalize those truths!

One of these fundamentals is the very concept of change. When we're children, our lives are full of changes, many of which occur because we don't control our environment, and others merely because of our age. We change from grade to grade, sometimes home to home. Our bodies change, our interests change, our friends change. As children, we're used to change. As adults, we can be more resistant. After all, we have more control over our environment and conclude, therefore, we should be more immune to change. As we hit forty and beyond, it can come as a shock when our bodies start to change—and not for the better! As adults, we must embrace the reality of the aging of our bodies but in a positive, proactive way. True, we can no longer be in our twenties again but forty-plus can still be a healthy, active, and vital time of life. We need to cultivate the belief that, while our bodies age, we can change and adapt for the better.

You've spent the first week gaining an awareness of the need for change. During this second week, I'd like you to focus on the benefits of change. One of the primary benefits is *longevity*. The statistics on the negative health impacts of carrying extra weight, having elevated cholesterol levels, living a sedentary life, or being under a stressful pressure cooker of events are undeniable. This type of lifestyle wears you down, wears you out, and inflates your weight. Over the years, these studies have marched a parade of bad news to anyone over forty.

There is good news, however! Studies show that even moderate changes to activity levels and eating patterns can reverse these negative impacts. A recent article in the *Dr. Julian Whitaker's Healing & Health* chronicled three separate studies on the benefits of moderate exercise.[1] So stick with it! Keep going. Be

1. Jakicic John M.; Bess H. Marcus; Kara I. Gallagher; Melissa Napolitano; Wei Lang. "Effect of Exercise Duration and Intensity on Weight Loss in Overweight, Sedentary Women: A Randomized Trial," *JAMA*, Vol. 290, No. 10 (2003): 1323–30 and McTiernan Anne; Charles Kooperberg; Emily White; Sara Wilcox; Ralph Coates; Lucile L. Adams-Campbell; Nancy Woods; Judith Ockene. "Recreational Physical Activity and the Risk of Breast Cancer in Postmenopausal Women: The Women's Health Initiative Cohort Study," *JAMA*, Vol. 290, No. 10 (2003): 1331–36 and Gregg Edward W., PhD; Robert B. Gerzoff, MS; Carl J. Caspersen, PhD; David F. Williamson, PhD; K. M. Venkat Narayan, MD. "Relationship of Walking to Mortality Among US Adults with Diabetes," *Arch Intern Med*, Vol. 163, No. 12 (2003): 1440–47

intentional this week about your eating, your drinking, and your physical activities.

For help increasing your level of physical activity, listen to the wise advice of Kenneth Cooper, M.D. Dr. Cooper is the founder of the Cooper Institute, a nonprofit research and education center founded in 1970 and recognized for its programs that focus on exercise physiology, behavior change, obesity, nutrition, aging, diabetes, hypertension, physical activity intervention, and health promotion (www.cooper aerobics.com). Dr. Cooper recommends the following steps for those over forty who have not been physically active but wish to begin a more intense exercise program:

- Get clearance from your primary-care physician, including having an electrocardiogram to determine how your heart will react.
- Go slowly and build your activity level to decrease the likelihood of injury or strain.
- Warm up properly through stretching. (Dr. Cooper recommends three to five minutes. Your stretching in the morning is an excellent way to do this!)
- Make sure to cool down gradually after exercise to allow your heart rate to return to normal before going into other tasks or activities.
- Track your heart rate during and after exercise to make sure you are not straining your heart. Your doctor can provide guidelines for target rates based upon your health.
- Engage in both aerobic and strength-training activities. (As a general guideline, Dr. Cooper recommends twenty to thirty minutes of aerobic exercise such as walking or jogging, at least three to five

as referenced in the November 2003 issue of Dr. Julian Whitaker's *Health & Healing* 13, No. 11, page 5.

times a week, and a twenty-minute strength-training activity at least twice a week.)
- Choose activities that match your physical condition.
- Listen to your body and don't ignore pain.

SUCCESS IN ACTION

This week, you'll face challenges in your resolve to maintain your commitment. Think over a typical week and write down in your journal three challenges you can expect to face. For one person they might be the latte on the morning drive, the box of doughnuts at work, the candy machine down the hall in the afternoon. Take time now, before they happen, to write down how you are going to overcome these challenges. For example, instead of a caffeine-laden pick-me-up on the way to work, how about opening a window and tuning in a favorite radio station or putting in a favorite tape or CD? If you enjoy it, sing loudly and with enthusiasm! I guarantee you'll feel pumped up and ready to go when you arrive! If you take a bus, train, or subway to work, why not engage a fellow passenger in conversation? Again, be creative and tailor the response to help you overcome the temptation.

WEEK 2   🦋   DAY 2

Today's Thin Thought: Don't underestimate the power of a dream.

Your daily assignments:
- **Drink lots of water.**
- **Bend, stretch, and move upon waking.**
- **Walk in the morning for at least fifteen minutes.**
- **Keep track of what you put in your mouth.**
- **Watch your servings.**

SETTING THE DAY FOR SUCCESS

Every great leap forward in your life comes after you've made a clear decision. In order to clarify your decision to be *Thin over* 40, I want you to try something. There's a concept in psychology called visualization. Athletes use this technique frequently to visualize victory. This allows them to remain upbeat and positive amid the rigors of physical and mental exertion. Today I want you to visualize what longevity and good health will mean to you in the future. Perhaps now you find it challenging to get out and walk for fifteen minutes. Go out and walk anyway. While you're out, visualize how you'll feel when you're able to walk twice that far without huffing and puffing or needing to stop periodically. Visualize how you'll feel when you've achieved your goal weight and are able to fit into smaller-sized clothing. Visualize your heart and circulatory system as you walk, able to operate without the strain of added weight and arterial buildup. Visualize being able to enjoy physical, even tiring, activities with family or friends, while still maintaining a good attitude.

When you find it hard to drink that water, visualize the water working through your system, cleansing your body. When confronted with a difficult choice about what to eat, visualize what that food item will do to your insides. Allow this mental image to dissuade you from eating the fatty, sugary item and motivate you to choose the healthy one. If you're tempted to go back for a second or third helping, visualize how it feels when you're so full you're uncomfortable. Then think about how good you'll feel if you leave yourself some room after eating.

So much of the changes you're making will be done through an internal dialogue. You must tell yourself over and over again why you are choosing to eat and act differently than you have in the past. Frankly, you may spend a portion of your time arguing with yourself. Be persistent. Keep reiterating your goals and desires. Visualize your success and your longevity.

SUCCESS IN ACTION

In your journal, write down three of your most powerful visualizations. These are, in essence, your dreams—your dreams of what you want to accomplish. Take the time to write them out in detail: what they mean to you, how you will feel, why they are so important. Then I want you to pick out a single phrase that you can use for each one. Write down each phrase and memorize it. You will use these as shields for times when you falter. Hopefully, they will keep you from stumbling, but if not, they can provide you the motivation to pick yourself back up and keep striving toward your dreams.

Realize that often our most powerful motivations for personal change come not from ourselves, but from others. Don't forget the positive effect your improved health can have on family, loved ones, and friends. I have known many clients who incorporated not only personal reasons for making healthy changes but also a desire to be healthy for spouses, beloved friends, children, and grandchildren. As I said before, it can be hard to change. Use all of your dreams to help point you in the right direction.

Now, some of you may think that dreaming is for dewy-eyed newlyweds or young kids. Don't buy into that false notion! Dreams are for everyone! With life being so busy through your twenties and thirties, it may have been quite a while since you sat down and really thought about your own personal dreams and goals. If it's good enough for fast-paced business managers and highly effective people, it's good enough for you! (For great motivation to dream and set goals, I heartily recommend *Timing is Everything: Turning Your Seasons of Success into Maximum Opportunities* by Denis Waitley.[2] This wonderful book is packed with helpful, commonsense strategies to incorporate your dreams and goals into everyday life, increasing your personal success. This information can be translated into many areas.) Acknowledge your dream of being *Thin over 40*. Allow your successes, wherever they may occur, to motivate you to continue to set goals for yourself.

WEEK 2 ❧ DAY 3

Today's Thin Thought: Two plus two equals four.

Your daily assignments:
- **Drink lots of water.**
- **Bend, stretch, and move upon waking.**
- **Walk in the morning for at least fifteen minutes.**
- **Keep track of what you put in your mouth.**
- **Watch your servings/portions.**

Your weekly assignment:
- **Weigh yourself.**

Don't be put off by getting on the scale. It's a way for you to measure your progress toward your goal weight. Remember, also, that you are less than two weeks into a long-term lifestyle change. The extra weight will come off, I promise you! What is more critical at this point, however, is for you to continue

2. Waitley, Denis. *Timing Is Everything: Turning Your Seasons of Success into Maximum Opportunities.* New York: Pocket Books, 1996.

with the Plan, recognizing that you're in it for the duration! Your success is about achieving your goals, but it's also about gaining the insight and understanding to support those goals. Be patient with yourself and keep at it!

SETTING THE DAY FOR SUCCESS

We are all governed by certain physical laws. Gravity. Entropy. Thermodynamics. We learned what they meant in school, but they've come to have a different meaning now that we're over forty. Gravity seems much more powerful as we look at the way our bodies have sagged over time. Entropy just points out how we seem to be falling apart more quickly than when we were younger. Thermodynamics means we aren't burning as many calories over forty as we were under twenty.

Some of us will look back on our younger days and be amazed at what behaviors we used to "get away" with—from overeating to overdrinking. We seemed to be able to live out an equation where two plus two did not always equal four. "Getting away with it" really was an illusion, two plus two really does equal four, and these excesses have a much longer shelf life in middle age than they did in our youth. Don't feel alone in this, however. Statistics show that Americans keep getting bigger and bigger each year, especially as our population ages. It seems increased weight has gone hand in hand with advancing age.

There are a variety of factors in this enlarging of the American populace, but I would like to focus on a major cause: Americans eat too much. Our concept of a typical meal today is quite different, quite a bit larger, than what it was even forty-five years ago. There was a fascinating article in the weekly national magazine, *U.S. News and World Report*, entitled "Supersize America: How Our Way of Life is Killing Us."[3] It compared foods from different time periods. What did it show? A hamburger in 1957 had 210 calories. In 2002, it had almost tripled, to 618. Movie popcorn in 1957 was 170 calories. By 2002, it was 900. In 1990, a Butterfinger candy bar had 270 calories, while in 2002, it had 680. In 1894, a bottle of Coca-Cola had 79 calories and today it has 250. The culprit? Larger amounts being sold as a single serving. In our minds, we have a 20-ounce pop and consider it a bottle of soda. Back when Coca-Cola started, a serving was considered 6.5 ounces, or a third as large. Yes, we've certainly bought into the philosophy that bigger is better. Except, bigger isn't better for our waistlines, now that we're over forty.

For the rest of this week, I'd like you to continue focusing on serving size and portion control. Use the information provided in the Food Guide Pyramid and on the back of packaging to determine the true size of a serving. Use that measurement to calculate the servings you eat. And continue your inner dialogue, because part of you will want to argue that the amount of food represented in a single serving is really not enough. After you've eaten your plateful, especially at your evening meal, wait five minutes before deciding whether or not you really want more. Give your stomach a chance to catch up with your mouth. You may find you're not really that hungry, after all. Your goal here is to begin to reorient your total food intake to more closely match the guidelines in the Food Guide Pyramid. (Later, we'll talk about personalizing those to your metabolic type. For now, go ahead and use this information as a general guide.)

3. Spake, Amanda with Mary Brophy Marcus. "A Fat Nation," 40, 41 *U.S. News & World Report*, August 19, 2002, pages 41–47.

You also want to continue tracking how much sodium, fats, carbohydrates, and calories you consume each day. Most people are carrying extra weight because of too many packaged foods, not an overabundance of broccoli in their diet. Your goal is to begin to reduce these amounts to get more in line with the recommended guidelines on the pyramid. This isn't the end of the process, but it is an excellent step toward greater health and longevity.

SUCCESS IN ACTION

All of us have a favorite restaurant and a favorite meal at that restaurant. In your journal, write down the restaurants you frequent and the meals you typically order. Look for any patterns. For example, do you typically eat ethnic food? Are your favorite selections fried or baked? Do you always order an appetizer and a dessert with your meal? How often do you go out? Include breakfast, lunch, and dinner.

Your assignment for today, or within the next few days, is to go to your favorite restaurant and order your favorite meal. If you get it as take-out, when you arrive home make sure to cut the meal in half and put half of it away in the refrigerator. If you are eating it at the restaurant, immediately ask for a box as soon as the item arrives. When the server brings you the box, cut the meal in half and put half in the box. Either way, enjoy the rest of your meal, making sure to drink your water before, during, and after. You now have lunch for the next day.

If your meal is like most meals served in restaurants today, the half portion you ate more closely resembles an actual single serving of that dish. Restaurants are notorious for large, generous portioning. By cutting it in half, you are allowing your favorite dish to give you enjoyment for two days, instead of one!

<h2 style="text-align:center">WEEK 2   🦋   DAY 4</h2>

Today's Thin Thought: Everything that goes in your mouth counts.

Your daily assignments:
- **Drink lots of water.**
- **Bend, stretch, and move upon waking.**
- **Walk in the morning for at least fifteen minutes.**
- **Keep track of what you put in your mouth.**
- **Watch your servings/portions.**

SETTING THE DAY FOR SUCCESS

The bane of every diet is the concept of counting calories. People just don't like the burden of tracking. The goal of *Thin over 40* is to free you from having to do that for the rest of your life. But in order to gain that freedom, you're going to need to spend a little bit of time tracking and, yes, counting your calories.

You've already gone a long way by keeping track of what you are eating in your food log in your journal. (If you've stopped doing this or didn't quite embrace this concept at the beginning with enthusiasm, please begin, begin again, or continue. It's important.) We'll talk later about each person's unique metabolism and what that means to you in terms of total caloric intake. For now, I want you to gain an understanding of how many calories you're consuming per day and per week and what those calories represent—protein, fats, or carbohydrates. Over the rest of this week, we are going to explore ways to cut down on that number of calories without entering into the den of starvation. We are also going to explore ways to exchange fat calories for protein or carbohydrate calories.

Why this fascination with calories? Because they represent what you are putting into your body. Again, you cannot change what you don't know. It is important to get a handle on the total amount of calories you consume each day and what those calories consist of. Let's look at how extra fat is accumulated on the body in two ways:

1. Through the overconsumption of fat calories in our daily caloric totals.

   Take a look at how many fat calories you are consuming and what percentage of your total calories those represent. The standard American diet today runs 40 percent or higher in fat calories. That's more fat than your body needs to carry on its necessary functions. The extra fat you eat ends up as the extra fat you carry.
2. Through a history of yo-yo dieting and caloric restriction.

   Every time you embark on a restrictive, low-calorie diet, it is initially successful. You lose weight. But at some point, your body adjusts to this starvation level by increasing production of an enzyme that determines how well the body stores fat. In other words, your body doesn't recognize you're just dieting, it thinks you're starving and revs up to make sure that every bit of fat you eat is immediately stored, not used. In addition, your metabolism slows down and you actually need less calories to carry on life than you did previously. Now, most people don't maintain this low-calorie diet for extended periods. Eventually, you get off the diet. But your body is still in the starvation mode, so when you return to a "normal" caloric intake, you gain your weight back more quickly and it gets converted more easily into fat.

SUCCESS IN ACTION

Get out your food logs and calculate the percentage of calories you are consuming as fat. How much should you eat in fats? The Food Guide Pyramid says you should eat no more than 30 percent of your calories as fat. If you eat 2,500 calories in a day, no more than 750 calories should be from fat. Most food labels list fat in grams, not calories. Each fat gram equals 9 calories. If you eat an item with 10 grams of fat per serving, each serving will have 90 calories of fat. In that same 2,500-calorie-per-day diet, the number of fat grams should be no more than 83.

Look over your food logs since you began tracking fat grams and determine the percentage of fat in your diet. Is it over 30 percent? If so, note those foods that represent the highest amount of fat. Can you eliminate one of the high-fat foods? Is it possible to have a smaller portion and reduce the fat? Write down three ways you can reduce the amount of fat you consume.

WEEK 2 ❦ DAY 5

Today's Thin Thought: Less can be more.

Your daily assignments:
- **Drink lots of water.**
- **Bend, stretch, and move upon waking.**
- **Walk in the morning for at least fifteen minutes.**
- **Keep track of what you put in your mouth.**
- **Watch your servings/portions.**
- **Watch your intake of unhealthy fats.**

How are you doing on your water, your stretching, and your walking? Just because we're going to be spending time focusing on the foods you eat does not mean you can slack off on the other aspects of the Plan. Remember, this is an integrated approach and each component supports the other!

SETTING THE DAY FOR SUCCESS

Some people have demonized fat. There are those who treat fat as a dirty word and vow to expunge any fat intake from their eating. This is dangerous and unhealthy. Our bodies need fat to function. The difficulty has been knowing which are good and which are bad types of fats we typically encounter. Let's go over the four types of fats:

1. saturated fats

   Found in red meat and some dairy products, as well as in some vegetable fat such as coconut, palm, and palm kernel oils.
2. polyunsaturated fats

   Found in safflower, flaxseed, sunflower, corn, soybean, and cottonseed oils. These types of fats are also found in some types of fish.
3. monounsaturated fats

   Found in olive, peanut, and canola oils.
4. trans fats or trans fatty acids

   Man-made fats found in prepared foods, such as cookies, cakes, doughnuts, crackers, French fries, and many frozen entrées. Trans fats are produced by the industrial process of hydrogenization—the adding of hydrogen to an oil to make it solid and more stable. When you look at ingredient labels and see the words "partially hydrogenated" or "hydrogenated" in front of a vegetable oil, you know that the product will contain trans fats. New labeling guidelines will soon require companies to list not only the amount of fat in foods but also to break down those fats into specific categories, such as saturated and trans fats.

Saturated fats are to be kept to a minimum. The Food Guide Pyramid recommends that no more than 30 percent of your total calories come from fat and, of those, not more than 10 percent should be saturated fats. In a 2,500 calorie per day diet, no more than 750 calories should come from fats and no more than 75 calories from saturated fats. Seventy-five calories is not very much. In order to help you track them, start differentiating in your daily food log how many grams of the fat you eat come from saturated fats. For example, if you eat a meal with 10 total grams of fat with 2 grams of saturated fats, note it as 10/2. For that meal, your saturated fat content was 20 percent of total fat, higher than recommended. These saturated fats can really catch up with you. There are some products naturally high in saturated fats, due to processing. Most baked goods like pastries, pies, cakes, and cookies are high in saturated fats. Therefore, these foods should be eaten sparingly. It doesn't mean you can't have them, just that you'll need to be careful how much.

But it's not always that simple, is it? These are often the very comfort foods we choose. For many, becoming an adult means finally getting to make your own choices about where you live, what you do with your time, and, yes, what you eat. Beginning as a young adult, you've been making choices about what you eat and what you drink. Now that you're forty and beyond, you're used to calling the nutritional shots. I won't try to tell you that changing those habits and choices is going to be easy. It's not, but it can become easier with knowledge and understanding.

You need to come a point where you love your body and your health more than you love that daily pastry or large bowl of ice cream every night. Often, these foods are eaten not because we are hungry but because we are accustomed to using them as relaxation or pleasure triggers. Our day at work might be stressful and chaotic, but we've come to look forward to that pastry or candy bar or (you fill in the blank) every day as a brief respite. At night, we've already eaten a large meal and our bodies have no real need for any more food, but our minds have come to anticipate that dessert as a "reward" at the end of a difficult day. We're going to work toward disconnecting this automatic response. Instead of choosing these foods just because you always have before, I want you to think about why you are eating them, what benefit they are to you, and whether or not you can choose to forego them altogether, eat less than you normally do, or substitute a healthier alternative.

SUCCESS IN ACTION

Look over your food logs and take note of times and places where you are eating high-fat high-calorie foods, apart from an established meal. Don't forget any beverages that are high calorie, like a milk shake, latte, or Frappuccino. Your goal is to give yourself permission to have these *less*. It doesn't mean you are giving them up forever, but rather you recognize that, while individually good, the amount you have been consuming is not contributing to good health or longevity. You will need to start consuming these items less frequently. Enjoy them fully when you do, but not as often. You're exchanging less of these foods for greater health.

WEEK 2 ✺ DAY 6

Today's Thin Thought: Ignorance is not bliss.

Your daily assignments:
- **Drink lots of water.**
- **Bend, stretch, and move upon waking.**
- **Walk in the morning for at least fifteen minutes.**
- **Keep track of what you put in your mouth.**
- **Watch your servings/portions.**
- **Watch your intake of unhealthy fats.**

Most of us have been too busy with life to really pay attention to all of this food tracking. It can seem cumbersome, but remember that you're not going to be doing this forever. You're concentrating on these things now so you can develop a natural habit of choosing healthy foods. You will get to the point where you will know how much of which foods you should be eating, and how often. But for right now, you need to invest the time in educating yourself about the foods you eat. Manufacturers don't always advertise the hidden amounts of fats, sugars, and sodium in their products. Their main concern is to sell products, not to promote your health. So, for now, it's up to you to keep a watchful eye.

Let's look at some ways you can cut down on the amount of fat you eat, even without reducing the amount of calories. Take, for example, that candy bar you have during the afternoon. It's just a regular-sized candy bar, say a Kit Kat bar. Pretty healthy, right? No nuts, just chocolate-covered vanilla sugar wafers. A Kit Kat bar has 290 calories. (For great information on nutritional breakdowns for many popular snack foods and desserts, go to www.uihc. uiowa.edu/fns/nutritional/vend.htm. Or you can go onto your Internet search engine and look up fat grams. This University of Iowa Web site is only one of many to provide detailed nutritional information on national brand products.)

Back to the Kit Kat bar. It has 290 calories, about the same number of calories as two fruit-and-grain bars. But a Kit Kat bar has 15 grams of fat, of which two-thirds, or 10 grams, are saturated fat. Two fruit-and-grain bars have 280 calories but 6 grams of fat, of which 17 percent, or 1 gram, is saturated fat. Let's look at it another way:

Item	Calories	Total Fat (grams)	Saturated Fat (grams)
Kit Kat bar	290	15	10
2 fruit-and-grain bars	280	6	1

For a medium-caloric intake of 2,200 calories per day, the current Food Guide Pyramid recommends no more than 73 total fat grams, of which no more than 24 grams should be saturated fat, consumed per day. By eating that one Kit Kat bar, you've just had more than 40 percent of your saturated fat and more than 20 percent of your total fat for the day. If you'd chosen to eat the two fruit-and-grain bars, you'd have eaten just 4 percent of your saturated fat and just 8 percent of your total fat. *All within the same amount of calories.*

Remember, when you eat more fat than you need, your body stores it. I'll never forget a card I once saw. It had a picture of doughnuts on the front, all kinds, with frosting and sprinkles. On the inside, the caption read: "For your birthday, a rare photo of hips in the larval stage." For those over forty, that card is more true than humorous. In order to be *Thin over 40*, you must begin a process of weaning yourself off excess unhealthy fats.

SUCCESS IN ACTION

Identify one comfort food you are willing to consume less of during this upcoming week. Write down why you've chosen this item and what you are going to remind yourself of to help you choose to forego it. Be positive with your answer. Concentrate on what you're gaining as opposed to what you're giving up. Tell yourself you're not giving it up forever but merely choosing to enjoy it less often. Remind yourself of the value of delayed gratification.

WEEK 2   🦋   DAY 7

Today's Thin Thought: Too much of a good thing can be bad.

Your daily assignments:
- **Drink lots of water.**
- **Bend, stretch, and move upon waking.**
- **Walk in the morning for at least fifteen minutes.**
- **Keep track of what you put in your mouth.**
- **Watch your servings/portions.**
- **Watch your intake of unhealthy fats.**

Weekly Assignment:
- Go grocery shopping for next week.

SETTING THE DAY FOR SUCCESS

Congratulations! You've come to the end of your second week. It's time to focus again on this week's Key Concept—Longevity. It may seem as if this week has been full of tracking calories and grams of this and that—and it has been. But the truth of the matter is that failing to track these things can have a serious and negative impact on your quality of life and your longevity. Too much of these things is bad for you. They increase your weight, elevate your blood pressure and your cholesterol, and compromise your health. Today I want you to use your maturity, gained through your years, to come to grips with the realization that you cannot continue to eat exactly as you have been. You can still eat all of the foods you like, just not in the *quantity* or *frequency*. That is reality. It's also the key to longevity. Of course, no one can predict how long any one person is going to live, but your chances of living longer, with a better quality of life, are enhanced by making these changes now.

Today, when you go out on your walk, I want you to have a serious talk with yourself about your health, your future, and what it is going to take to make these positive changes in your life. Be firm and committed to them. Talk to yourself and tell yourself these are good and right for you to do. Then listen, really listen, to what you hear back. You'll hear all of the built-up reasons and excuses for not wanting to change. Counter each and every one of them with a positive truth. We are talking about your life. We are talking about your health. Try to look at this as embracing a new, exciting way of eating. I promise that you will feel better. You'll have increased energy and vitality.

Success in Action

Before you go grocery shopping today, take some time to look over your comfort foods and formulate alternatives. Like the example given, choose a fruit-and-grain bar over your normal candy bar. Bring an apple or orange to work to eat, while everyone else is having a pastry. Instead of a large bowl of ice cream after dinner, try a small container of nonfat yogurt with fruit. Don't deprive yourself, just choose to treat yourself in a different way, with something healthy. Your body will thank you! Make sure to put these choices on your shopping list. That way, the alternative is ready to go when temptation strikes!

Keep drinking your water. Keep stretching. Keep walking. Keep educating yourself on what you're eating. Keep examining why you're eating what you eat. Keep committing to making the healthy changes you *know* will add vitality and longevity to your life!

Hero of the Week

This week, I want you to hear about Elaine, from Elaine:

> I told myself I was just meant to be heavy. It ran in the family. My mother was heavy. I figured we were just doomed to obesity in my family. The best we could do was hide our weight and go on. I hated my body. Because I hated it, I used it as little as possible. I never walked anywhere. Never climbed stairs. Never enjoyed any physical activity. Didn't even

like to be outside because it always involved movement of some sort.

It wasn't easy for Elaine to turn her life around. A
family history of obesity centered around an extremely high-fat food selection and preparation. She
grew up with a steady diet of fatty foods—from fried
eggs and bacon in the morning to battered-and-fried
vegetables and meat cuts for lunch and dinner. Her
mother's kitchen was constantly full of popping and
sizzling fat, and Elaine repeated that pattern into her
adulthood. The larger she grew, the more she came
to hate her body. The larger she grew, the greater
the temptation to blame genetics, while overlooking
other factors.

In order for Elaine to change, she needed to feel
differently about herself and then she needed to feed
herself differently. She needed to learn that she
wasn't born to be heavy. Slowly, Elaine came to
terms with her faulty conclusions and her self-hatred
regarding her weight and her body. As her perceptions changed, she was able to let go of family eating
patterns and adopt new, healthy ones.

Today Elaine lives an active, *Thin over 40* lifestyle.
She has learned to love her body, to move her body,
and to realize she isn't condemned by genetics or
family patterns to die young like her mother. Elaine
is my Hero of the Week because she has chosen to
strive for her own longevity!

WEEK 3
MAKING THE MOST OF MOVING

WEEK 3 🦋 DAY 1

Today's Thin Thought: Exercise is not a dirty word.

Welcome to your third week of *Thin over 40*! Keep going. You are setting the stage for lifelong changes that will enhance your health, your outlook, and your life. You need to keep with it and continually remind yourself how important this is. You've come a long way so far and I want you to stay with your excellent progress! Continue to do the following:

Your daily assignments:
- **Drink lots of water.** Keep water with you at all times and take sips periodically. This will help you stay hydrated during the day.
- **Bend, stretch, and move upon waking.** Don't skimp on this meaningful activity. Your body will thank you!
- **Walk in the morning for at least twenty minutes.** Yes, five more minutes—you can do it!
- **Keep track of what you put in your mouth.** Be aware of what you eat and avoid the unwanted calories of distracted eating.
- **Watch your servings/portions.** Keep telling yourself you can do with less. Give your stomach time to catch up at meals.

- **Watch your intake of unhealthy fats.** Watch for those saturated fats and trans fatty acids.

SETTING THE DAY FOR SUCCESS

The Key Concept for this week is Metabolism. Metabolism is simply the rate at which our bodies burn calories, whether we are resting or active. As our bodies age, our metabolism slows down. Fewer of the calories we eat are utilized to fuel our bodies and a greater percentage is stored as fat. We slow down and get larger. The larger we get, the more challenging it is to get up and move at all. The bigger we are, the less we move. The less we move, the bigger we get. This is the vicious cycle of middle age.

The good news is we are able to speed up our metabolism. This week, we will concentrate on the first of four ways to boost metabolism—exercise. Some of you will look at that word and conjure up a negative image of aching muscles, labored breath, and sweat-stained shirts. The whole idea is repugnant to you. You just want to lose some weight, not look like Arnold Schwarzenegger. (If you're thinking that way, relax—none of us will ever look like Arnold Schwarzenegger!) But you can utilize exercise and increased physical movement to help ratchet up your metabolic rates. As a bonus, you'll increase your lean muscle mass, reduce excess fat, look better, and *feel* better.

You are already well on your way to increasing your metabolism by developing your habit of moving and walking upon waking. This habit, which jump-starts your metabolic rate in the morning, lasts into the day. This week and next, I want you to increase your walking time from fifteen minutes to twenty minutes. It's only five minutes more! Hopefully, by this third week, you've come to appreciate and anticipate this special time just for you. No phones, no faxes, no questions from others, no agendas beyond just getting out, moving your body, and preparing yourself mentally, and metabolically, for the day. If you experience any pain from walking, it might be beneficial to visit a custom orthodics store. Orthodics is just a fancy name for foot pads or supports. As we age, and especially if we're carrying a large amount of excess weight, the bones in our feet can misalign and produce pain, not only in our feet but also in our backs, knees, and joints. If this is the case for you, and you're not sure you are able to increase the amount of time you walk, I encourage you to look into obtaining custom orthodics and/or shoes, designed to support your weight and reduce the strain on your feet. You'll walk more if it hurts less.

Getting out and moving your body can be done all through the day, in addition to your special time in the morning. This week, we'll look at ways you can increase the amount of your physical movement as a natural part of the day. We'll also continue to look at ways to integrate healthy eating habits.

All of this must be motivated, in part, by a genuine love and appreciation for your body. If you don't love your body, you have no reason to feed or move it properly. Many of you are ashamed of your bodies, how they look and how they move. You cover them up with baggy clothing. You look at yourself in the mirror with disgust. You unfavorably compare what you're able to do now with what you were able to do when you were younger. You hate getting older and you hate what it's doing to your body.

Stop thinking this is a permanent condition. It is not! Even over the past two weeks, you've seen improvement. Your body, over forty though it is, is still able to respond to your intentional lifestyle changes in a positive way. Studies demonstrate the body's ability to build muscle and lose fat through exercise even into your eighties. So enough excuses! It's time to get moving!

SUCCESS IN ACTION

In your journal, write down three things you like about your body. If you have trouble coming up with three, this is a clue to how your attitude has gotten warped over the years! Write a commitment to your body to continue making positive changes to improve your physical condition and your health.

Your assignment today is to obtain a set of low-weight barbells. You are going to begin integrating the use of these barbells during your time of stretching in the morning. Go ahead and continue to do your normal stretching, but use these barbells to add some load to what you are asking your muscles to do. Remember to stretch and extend slowly and completely, paying attention to how your muscles are feeling. When walking, you use your lower-body muscles. By adding these weights, you'll be working your upper body—arms, back, and shoulders.

In choosing the weights, think lighter rather than heavier. Your goal is not to choose the heaviest weight you can pick up. Instead, you want a lighter weight so you'll be able to do a greater number of repetitions. Low weight—lots of reps. A weight that you're barely able to lift five times is too heavy. If you can lift it fifteen or more times without noticeable effort, it's too light. You're looking for a weight that you can lift without straining initially, but by ten to fifteen reps, you are feeling the tension. The goal is not to accomplish these lifts quickly or with a jerking motion. Rather, these lifts are to be done slowly, concentrating on the specific motion involved. Many people make the mistake of "heaving" a weight in order to lift it. It takes sustained effort to slowly lift the weight up and down in the proper position, not cheating by creating momentum through speed. If you have a question, ask a salesperson to assist you in choosing a weight range that works for you. The larger athletic equipment stores will have samples available for you to try out before you buy. Don't be embarrassed to ask for help! You'll avoid injury strains and build endurance. Again, the goal is not to look like a bodybuilder but to build up your body and increase the amount of muscle tissue you have. Muscle tissue acts as a furnace for burning calories. The more muscle tissue you have, the higher your metabolic rate, even when you're resting. A little strength work in the morning will help you burn more calories, even if you sit in a chair all day long! (Hold that thought, we'll explore it more tomorrow!)

WEEK 3 ❦ DAY 2

Today's Thin Thought: There's more to your workday than a desk.

Your daily assignments:
- Drink lots of water.
- Bend, stretch, and move upon waking.
- Walk in the morning for at least twenty minutes.
- Keep track of what you put in your mouth.
- Watch your servings/portions.
- Watch your intake of unhealthy fats.
- Move more during the day.

SETTING THE DAY FOR SUCCESS

The bane of metabolism is our sedentary lifestyles. We don't move enough. We sit at a desk all day or we're in the car far too much. At forty and beyond, we look for ways to sit whenever possible, because we're tired and our feet hurt. In addition, many of us are at that place in our careers where sitting at a desk or talking on the phone is the bulk of our daily activity. Some of you may spend a great deal of time sitting and driving. The common thread is sitting, which isn't really an activity at all. It is, however, a reality in your day that must be factored into your *Thin over 40* lifestyle.

Our bodies do much better when we get up periodically and move around. Many of us spend a great deal of time looking at a computer screen. This kind of focused concentration can produce great results as far as work product is concerned, but it also produces eye, neck, and back strain. Studies on repetitive injuries in the workplace recommend a change in position every so often, just to break up the stress on those muscles. I heartily agree! This week I want you to look for ways you can get up and move around at work, as an intentional part of your day. Here are just a few good reasons why:

- To reduce eye and muscle strain from remaining in a fixed position.
- To take a break from intense concentration to give yourself a mental pause.
- To allow for increased circulation throughout your body. When we sit, areas such as legs and feet can experience diminished blood flow.
- To intentionally replace eating at your desk as a way to "take a break."
- To relieve stress.

Let's face it, many of us are in high-stress jobs, either because of the type of work we do or because we're being asked to do more and more at work with less time to do it. Worker productivity is at an all-time high because fewer numbers of workers are handling the same amount of work or more. Americans are working longer hours with one of the smallest percentages of vacation time for any industrialized nation. This produces a great deal of stress, and we have come to use food as a way to relieve that stress, both at home and at work. It's time to make some changes in how we handle stress and do it in such a way that contributes to a healthy metabolism instead of solidifying a sedentary lifestyle.

SUCCESS IN ACTION

In your journal, write down how you deal with stress at work and why. Really think over the course of your workday and write down every strategy, from snacking to tensing your back to barking orders at others to working nonstop without a break. At the end of the day, how do you feel? Are you relaxed and feeling confident about the day, or do you just want to get home and forget it all? Do you feel good about yourself and what you've been able to accomplish, or do you beat yourself up for not doing enough? How you feel about yourself at work can often determine how you choose to de-stress once you're home. (Again, hold that thought—we'll talk about it tomorrow.)

At work today I want you to get up and take a moving break—not an eating break—three times during your day. Get up once in midmorning and walk around the building, the plant, the office, the block—just for a couple of minutes. Even if you are still inside, get away from your immediate work environment. You want to be able to breathe deep, stretch your legs, even move your arms. The goal is to disperse that stress you've been building up, both mental and physical. Take your water with you and use this time to rehydrate. This is the kind of break your body needs!

Remember, work is to be a no-snack zone, and you're only to eat when you're truly hungry and ready for a meal. After your meal today, make sure you get up and take another physical break. Your third break should come in the later afternoon (or if you're on shift work, about an hour or so prior to the end of your shift). This can be a natural "low" time, when the temptation to grab a snack or a soda is high. Years ago, the soft drink Dr Pepper used to have a clock on the bottle with the numbers ten, two, and four highlighted. These were the times you were supposed to take a break from your day and have a Dr Pepper. While drinking a calorie-laden beverage three times a day isn't a great idea, taking a break at regular intervals is. Analyze your work flow and figure out two additional times to get up this week, along with right after you eat your lunch or equivalent meal, one toward the beginning of your shift and one toward the end. You'll be amazed at how refreshing these times can be and how much your stress level during the day can de-escalate. You'll feel better and work better.

WEEK 3 🦋 DAY 3

Today's Thin Thought: Stress is a drag, but exercise is a lift.

Your daily assignments:
- **Drink lots of water.**

- Bend, stretch, and move upon waking.
- Walk in the morning for at least twenty minutes.
- Keep track of what you put in your mouth.
- Watch your servings/portions.
- Watch your intake of unhealthy fats.
- Move more during the day.

Your weekly assignment:
- Weigh yourself.

SETTING THE DAY FOR SUCCESS

Increased physical movement not only increases our metabolism, it also decreases our stress. Stress is a real drag on metabolism. When we're stressed, we tend to eat to cope. This excess weight slows us down and reduces our metabolism. Stress also makes us weary, with some of us too tired to even move out of our easy chairs or off of the couch when we get home at the end of the day. Stress saps our strength, our energy, our enthusiasm for life. It can also produce significant health problems that slow us down further.

One of the fundamental changes you need to make is in how you deal with the stress in your life. I would like to offer increased physical movement as a healthy, realistic coping mechanism. Consider replacing "moving time" for "food time" as your downtime. What that means is making sure that you engage in some level of physical activity at the end of your day as a healthy way to unwind and de-stress.

This doesn't mean going out and jogging after dinner. What it does mean is making sure that you aren't just sitting down from the time you scoot your chair in after dinner to the time you get up to go to bed in the evening. For most people, this span of time can be anywhere from three to five hours. A few minutes relaxing is great, but a pattern of sedentary behavior night after night, after a full day of sitting or minimal activity at work, does nothing to reverse your body's natural tendency to slow down your metabolism as you age. Early evening needs to return to a time of family, friends, and meaningful activities instead of reclining in your chair waiting to go to bed. Here are a few ways you can increase your physical activity level and make the most of this time (you will probably have better long-term results if you choose a variety of activities to engage in):

- Take a walk with a family member, a friend, or your dog. (If you're concerned this is too much walking with the twenty minutes you're doing in the morning, please realize that the current guidelines for adults is *sixty minutes* of physical activity per day.)
- Take a weekly class at a community center, community college, or activity center, such as ballroom dancing, square dancing, yoga, even belly dancing!
- Plan a date night with your spouse or partner to meet for dinner and a walk around a favorite neighborhood or park, or along a beach or lake.
- Play an outdoor game with your children, either in your yard, a park, or a school playfield.
- Go to the local community pool. Many have specific water exercise classes you can take in the evenings. Water acts as a cushion, which is great for those with joint difficulties.
- Join a club tailored to your fitness level, where you can go a couple of times a week to engage in exercises designed to strengthen and work needed areas, such as knees, backs, or arms. Trust me, not

every fitness center is meant for slim singles. Check with your city recreation center. Many have exercise facilities factored with all ages and ability levels in mind. Another advantage is that you should be able to pay per visit, as opposed to having to buy a membership like at for-profit fitness clubs.

- Get outside and do a little work in your yard or garden.

These are just suggestions. Depending upon your situation, you may need to be creative in finding a solution to the couch-potato syndrome. Whenever possible, involve someone else with you. On the days you feel unmotivated, their companionship could be just what you need to get you over the hump.

SUCCESS IN ACTION

In your journal, list three alternate activities you are going to engage in the rest of this week during your evening hours (or equivalent downtime). Be specific and list what you will do, when you will do them, and anyone you want to participate with you in them. If you need to plan ahead, write down what you'll need to do and when you'll need to do it by. This is intentional planning. So often, if we don't have things planned, we'll opt for what we usually do, which for many can be nothing. Make sure to tailor your activities to where you are right now physically. You do not want to do something too strenuous and risk injury. Remember, you're a turtle, building habits for life, not a rabbit, scampering toward some short-term goal! Slow and steady wins the race. Baby steps at first lead to great strides over the long term.

WEEK 3   🦋   DAY 4

*Today's Thin Thought: It's better to go to bed
a little empty than too full.*

Your daily assignments:
- Drink lots of water.
- Bend, stretch, and move upon waking.
- Walk in the morning for at least twenty
  minutes.
- Keep track of what you put in your mouth.
- Watch your servings/portions.
- Watch your intake of unhealthy fats.
- Move more during the day.

SETTING THE DAY FOR SUCCESS

To start off today, we're actually going to talk
about tonight. For many people, their real danger
zone becomes not merely a place—their own
kitchens—but also a time—the evening hours. Recently, the American Psychological Association made
a modification to the eating disorders category to include nighttime binge eating. It seems that a percentage of people struggle under a compulsion to eat
more than is needed during the evening hours. During my work with eating disorders, I have certainly
seen this to be true. There is something about the
evening, the time we unwind, and a kitchen full of
food, that can present people with a desire to eat
well beyond full.

Ideally, you want to consume the bulk of your calories before 3:00 p.m. in the afternoon. This way,
your stomach will be relatively empty during sleep.
How many of us have overeaten an evening meal or
indulged in too large a late-night snack and then
found it difficult to relax and go to sleep? Overeating

at night also causes your insulin levels to surge, prompting the familiar drowsiness after dinner. The more you eat, the more energy your body puts into the digestive process, and the less energy you have to get up, get out, and get moving.

Today I want you to intentionally eat a smaller, lighter meal at dinner. Get up from the table after one serving, instead of eating your way through two or three, and have more time to relax, to enjoy your family or favorite book. Be intentional about the amount of food you put on your plate, and get up as soon as you are through. Make sure to drink your water throughout dinner. (I have heard it said that you shouldn't drink water during your meal because this can interfere with your stomach's ability to digest the food you eat. Relax, and drink your water! The digestive acids in your stomach are not compromised by water consumption. Water actually aids in digestion. So drink all you want!)

Remember, your goal is to increase the amount of physical activity you do throughout the day and evening, in order to boost your metabolism. You'll feel more energetic and optimistic. Heavy, caloric meals in the evening only contribute to your desire to snooze away the evening before you head to bed! Think light—think active—think interactive—for your evening hours!

SUCCESS IN ACTION

In your journal today, write two ways you tend to overeat at night. It could be waiting too late to have dinner and then eating everything in sight. It could be your ritual of a bowl of ice cream about an hour after dinner. Or it could be the package of cookies or candy you keep on hand for "just a snack" before you go to bed. Do you have some special concoction you make regularly? Identify what you eat and why you find that meaningful and comforting. Brainstorm ways you can substitute a different activity. Perhaps it will be reading a book or saving a special section of the paper to read or brewing up a hot cup of tea or sugar-free hot chocolate. Be prepared to make an active change in your evening pattern.

WEEK 3   🦋   DAY 5

Today's Thin Thought: Many small steps add up to giant leaps.

Your daily assignments:
- **Drink lots of water.**
- **Bend, stretch, and move upon waking.**
- **Walk in the morning for at least twenty minutes.**
- **Keep track of what you put in your mouth.**
- **Watch your servings/portions.**
- **Watch your intake of unhealthy fats.**
- **Move more during the day.**

SETTING THE DAY FOR SUCCESS

We live in a convenient society, with transportation systems to take us to all our destinations. We live in an accelerated society, where speed trumps just about everything. We've gotten used to driving around at the store for twenty minutes in order to find a closer parking spot. High-rise buildings have express elevators to avoid the time-consuming possibility of too many people wanting in on too many floors. Efficiency equates with speed. If it's done quickly, it's done well.

The problem with our efficient society is we've designed out the component of people getting themselves where they need to go. We've factored out a good deal of the built-in physical activity of many functions. As you continue to incorporate *Thin over 40* habits, I want you to look for ways to reintroduce physical activity into your day.

Allow me to offer you some suggestions. These are not meant as a checklist, but rather as a way to stimulate your own imagination as you think over your day and how you can incorporate more movement:

- If you drive to work, park farther away from your building and walk. Be sure to factor in some extra time to do this so you won't add to your stress by being late!
- If you take a bus or subway, try getting out at an earlier stop and walk the rest of the way to your destination.
- Once you're at work, consider using the stairs instead of the elevator. If you're on the thirty-seventh floor, start out by walking the first two floors and taking the elevator the rest of the way. As your physical condition improves, work toward increasing the number of stairs you walk versus the number of floors you ride the elevator.
- Instead of always asking other workers or subordinates to obtain needed items, stand up and use the opportunity to stretch a little on your way, and get that item for yourself.
- Whenever possible, use the stairs instead of escalators at stores or buildings.
- If you're going shopping at a particular store at the mall, park at the opposite end and walk there and back.
- If you're going to be doing a variety of errands in a central location, park your car in the middle and

walk from store to store instead of driving to each one.

- If you need to speak with a coworker, walk down the hall to his or her office instead of picking up the phone.
- If you have a cell phone, plan to place some of your calls as you are taking a walk around the block. Take care of business and your health, all at the same time!

By achieving a higher activity level during the day, you help your metabolism maintain a corresponding higher rate. The higher your metabolism, the more calories you burn. You feel more alert, your mood is more optimistic; you're less tired and cold.

SUCCESS IN ACTION

Think about your day and plan two concrete ways to increase your activity level as a natural part of your routine. Calculate the extra time needed to get yourself where you need to go, as opposed to being transported there in some way. Give yourself permission to use that time for your own health and well-being.

WEEK 3 🦋 DAY 6

Today's Thin Thought: An ounce of prevention is worth a pound of cure.

Your daily assignments:
- **Drink lots of water.**
- **Bend, stretch, and move upon waking.**
- **Walk in the morning for at least twenty minutes.**
- **Keep track of what you put in your mouth.**
- **Watch your servings/portions.**

- Watch your intake of unhealthy fats.
- Move more during the day.

My thanks to Benjamin Franklin for today's Thin Thought!

Getting up and moving as a part of your day can, at first, seem forced and unnatural. It can seem a waste of time. Consider, however, that this small increase—these baby steps—lead to increased physical fitness that can allow you to do even more. Will your muscles ache now and again? Yes, but this is merely your body adjusting to your increased physical demands. It will respond!

Consider, also, the alternative. If you stay on a course of becoming more and more sedentary—while becoming larger and larger—your body will also respond, and not in a positive way. Excess weight puts a tremendous strain on muscles and joints, to say nothing of major organs like your heart. Your daily increased movement is your ounce of prevention.

If today is your weekend, you have a wonderful opportunity to evaluate how you are going to use this day. I encourage you to choose an activity today that will give you a great deal of pleasure, as well as get you out and get you moving. Your goal is to work your heart and your muscles by exceeding the level you've reached during the week. Physical conditioning is gained through gently stretching your limits. Go on a longer walk or do your same walk faster. Do an extra set of stretches today with your weights. If you're used to walking relatively flat stretches, find a different neighborhood or setting that has a series of hills. If you need inspiration and are able, go out and play with your children. Their energy and enthusiasm will be sure to test your limits!

SUCCESS IN ACTION

By getting up and increasing your movement, you run counter to established routines and habits that have had 40-plus years to take hold. In order to counter those habits, I want you to come up with two positive affirmation statements that you can repeat to yourself during the day. Here are some examples to help you create your own:

> "My mind is free to think when my body is free to move."
> "Getting up and moving helps me get more from my day."
> "I release my stress when I get up and move."
> "A sedentary lifestyle is a waste of my time."

WEEK 3   🦋   DAY 7

Today's Thin Thought: Health comes through a change in lifestyle, not obsession.

Your daily assignments:
• Drink lots of water.
• Bend, stretch, and move upon waking.
• Walk in the morning for at least twenty minutes.
• Keep track of what you put in your mouth.
• Watch your servings/portions.
• Watch your intake of unhealthy fats.
• Move more during the day.

Weekly Assignment:
• Go grocery shopping for next week.

Amazing! You've been sticking with the Plan for three weeks now! You're taking the steps necessary to integrate these changes as a regular part of your life. I cannot encourage you enough to keep going, keep staying the course. Be optimistic and upbeat about your success and the future. If you've found yourself faltering a bit, recommit to extra effort next week. Keep taking those baby steps and you'll be amazed how far you'll travel!

SETTING THE DAY FOR SUCCESS

I want you to take some time today and think back over the course of your week, and the ways you've already increased your activity and decreased your stress level. I promise you that if you will keep at it, these benefits are only the beginning! And I'd like you to focus today on the benefits, not on the behaviors. In my treatment of those with eating disorders, I have seen the distortion that can take place when people focus on what they are doing as opposed to why. The goal of increased movement is for you to experience the refreshment available when you use your body in a more active way. The why is for you to feel more energized, relaxed, and healthy. It does not make you more virtuous to walk across a parking lot instead of parking right next to the door. You have no greater claim to superiority because you take the stairs at work instead of getting into the elevator. Rather, these are actions you have chosen to do because they make *you* feel better. This isn't about anyone else—it's about you. As you are working toward developing these new habits, please integrate them into a balanced lifestyle and attitude. This isn't about obsession or rituals; it's about an active, positive mind-set.

With that in mind, I want to remind you today, as we've spent the week thinking about physical movement and exercise, of the importance of rest. Our bodies also need time to rest, especially if you stretched yourself yesterday. Resting at the end of an active week is quite different from an ongoing pattern of nonactivity. It's okay to give yourself permission to rest because it's purposeful and short in duration.

Now, you are still going to be stretching upon waking and doing your walking. These are essentials in your day. But it is fine for you to take a day during the week to allow your body a chance to catch up to your increased activity level. This will allow your muscles, in particular, a chance to do some rebuilding. As they rebuild, they strengthen so you'll be ready for next week. Be sure to drink your water and continue your healthy eating. These will give your body the elements it needs to rejuvenate and rebuild.

SUCCESS IN ACTION

As you are choosing your meals for next week, be thinking about how your choices will affect your ability to get out and move. Will the foods you've chosen tend to weigh you down? Have you included plenty of fresh fruits and vegetables to give your body the vitamins it needs to operate properly? Have you included a good selection of lean meats, high in protein? Remember to think of your food as fuel for your healthy lifestyle.

In your journal today, I want you to write about how the week has gone. Be candid about the struggles you've faced as you've worked toward increasing your physical activity level. Write down the negative thoughts that have come to your mind as excuses for not following through during the day with what you've planned in the morning. Look at just one of these struggles and develop a way to get around that roadblock next week. Be positive and optimistic about your ability to overcome that obstacle. Write down how you look forward to the week ahead and the continued progress you'll be making.

HERO OF THE WEEK

I'd like you to take inspiration this week from a wonderful woman named Victoria Johnson. I first became acquainted with her because of her book, *Body Revival*. In it, Victoria chronicles her own journey from obesity to vibrant health. (For more information about Victoria, please check out her Web site at www.victoriajohnson.com.) Victoria says, "Don't work out for how it makes you look; work out for how it makes you feel, because exercise means ENERGY and a longer life, which is the bottom line." Victoria has overcome a lifetime of eating disorders and obesity to become an inspiration for those seeking to increase the level of exercise and movement in their lives. Believe me when I say she is an absolute joy and a bundle of boundless energy! For her optimism and belief in the ability to change for the better, Victoria Johnson is my Hero of the Week!

WEEK 4
MAKING THE MOST OF NUTRITION

WEEK 4 🦋 DAY 1

Today's Thin Thought: What you eat affects how you feel.

Welcome to your fourth week of *Thin over 40*! Each day you are taking the steps needed to anchor yourself to this healthy, rejuvenating lifestyle. Now is not the time to think you've got this thing figured out. Now is not the time to pick and choose what you will or won't do. Now is not the time to slack off. Now is the time to recommit yourself to the *Thin over 40* Plan and keep up with the changes you know are contributing to increased health and longevity!

Your daily assignments:
- Drink lots of water.
- Bend, stretch, and move upon waking.
- Walk in the morning for at least twenty minutes.
- Keep track of what you put in your mouth.
- Watch your servings/portions.
- Watch your intake of unhealthy fats.
- Move more during the day.

SETTING THE DAY FOR SUCCESS

The Key Concept for this week is Food and Mood. What you eat really does affect how you feel. And part of that difference has to do with the way the foods you eat affect your metabolism. When you feel run down, sluggish, unenergetic, you tend to have a depressed mood. You don't feel good and your attitude reflects that.

Metabolism, the rate at which you burn calories, is like the heat of a fire. A hot, active fire burns fuel more quickly, while a slower, cooler fire takes longer to burn fuel and does not burn it as efficiently. You want your metabolism to be a hot, active fire that takes what you eat, utilizes it, and leaves less fuel to be converted into fat by the body. The fuel or food you use can affect how hot your fire burns.

Today, many of the foods we eat are highly processed. They are full of refined sugar that enters the bloodstream on a fast track. On the surface, it would seem that these kinds of foods would be the perfect fuel to stoke up your metabolic fire. On the contrary, these foods do the exact opposite. These fragmented foods supercharge your system by spiking your blood sugar, or glucose, levels. They don't require a hot, active fire to burn because they are already so broken down in processing, they can enter your bloodstream almost immediately.

Once your blood-sugar level has been elevated, your body responds by producing insulin. Insulin takes the excess sugar or glucose in your blood and stores in it your cells as fat. When you eat highly refined foods, high in sugar, you are setting yourself up for a roller-coaster ride of glucose and insulin. Your glucose levels spike, so insulin rushes in to counterbalance it. But if there is an overabundance of insulin produced, it not only takes the glucose and stores it away as fat, it also leaves too little in your blood to be used. This drop in blood-sugar level causes fatigue and intense cravings, usually for those

foods high in carbohydrates, which can be easily converted into glucose by the body.

You get hungry and eat. But shortly after, you feel
tired, and not too long after that, you're craving
sweets or carbohydrates to feel better. So you get
hungry and eat again. These peaks and valleys can
cause a person to go over the edge into binge eating.
Through all of these highs and lows of your blood
sugar, there is a corresponding roller coaster of
your moods.

Believe me, there is a better way!

Instead of highly processed, fragmented foods, you
want to begin to substitute whole foods in your meal
planning. Whole foods, such as fresh fruits and vegetables, whole grains, and beans, take longer to be
digested. As such, the amount of sugars/carbohy-
drates is released over a longer period of time. You
avoid the spikes of blood sugar and the corresponding overproduction of insulin that causes the Jekyll
and Hyde effect. When foods take longer to digest,
they require your body to work harder. You are basically using calories to gain calories. This keeps your
metabolism higher, your fire hot and active.

SUCCESS IN ACTION

I want you to take this week to record in your
journal how you feel after each meal. Do you feel
energized and refreshed after eating, or do you feel
weighed down and lethargic? Do you experience
cravings within an hour after you eat? Two hours
after you eat? If you do experience cravings, write
down the first food that comes to mind. What is it
you're wanting? Is this a common desire? Start to
become more aware of how what you eat affects how
you feel. We'll continue working this week on substi-

tuting whole foods for highly processed or fragmented ones.

WEEK 4 🦋 DAY 2

Today's Thin Thought: An apple a day keeps the doctor away.

Your daily assignments:
- **Drink lots of water.**
- **Bend, stretch, and move upon waking.**
- **Walk in the morning for at least twenty minutes.**
- **Keep track of what you put in your mouth.**
- **Watch your servings/portions.**
- **Watch your intake of unhealthy fats.**
- **Move more during the day.**
- **Choose whole foods over fragmented foods.**

SETTING THE DAY FOR SUCCESS

Part of what we're talking about this week falls under the category of Glycemic Index. Originally, this concept arose as a way to help diabetics manage their daily blood sugar and, thereby, their need for insulin. It used to be thought that diabetics needed to avoid only sugar, since sugar caused their blood-sugar levels to rise too rapidly. The common wisdom was that carbohydrates could be eaten without difficulty, as they were assimilated into the bloodstream more slowly, avoiding a sugar spike. Diabetic researchers decided to test this theory about how quickly certain foods sent sugar into the bloodstream. Using either sugar itself or white bread as a baseline measure of 100, they tested how quickly 50 grams of food turned to sugar in the blood and called the resulting number its Glycemic Index. Foods that break down slowly, raising blood sugar slowly, have lower glycemic indexes than foods that break down readily.

This concept was quite revolutionary when it came out in 1999. There was a problem with it, however. Carrots have a GI of 131, while sugar has a GI of 100. This would seem to imply that, going by the Glycemic Index, sugar is better for you than carrots. Of course, we know that's not right! So how did the innocent carrot receive such a high GI? Remember that the GI was based on how fast 50 grams of a specific food turned into sugar in the bloodstream; the average serving of carrots has only 4 grams of carbohydrates. In other words, the GI for carrots was based on a serving of over one and a half pounds of carrots!

Fixing this problem with the Glycemic Index led to the concept of "Glycemic Load." The Glycemic Load takes the Glycemic Index of a food and multiplies it by the number of carbohydrates in a serving. In the case of the carrot, the GI of 131 is represented as 1.31, which is then multiplied by 4, the number of grams per serving. This equals 5.24, so carrots have a Glycemic *Index* of 131 but a Glycemic *Load* of about 5.

Did I mention there was also a problem with the Glycemic Load? Under the GI, 50 grams of ice cream has a rating of 37. Its GL is 4. So, ice cream has a better (lower) GL than carrots. But 50 grams of ice cream is around a third of a cup. Most of us don't eat just a third of a cup of ice cream—a typical serving size is a half cup, and many of us eat twice that in a sitting!

If all of this makes you feel like you've gone back to middle-school math, relax, there isn't going to be a test. This research merely points out the benefits of eating whole foods and avoiding an overabundance of processed, refined foods. The higher the processing, the quicker it floods into your system. The more "whole" the food, the longer it takes to digest, with its husk and skin and fiber. Thinking "whole foods" is a lot easier to remember and use as you make choices every day.

SUCCESS IN ACTION

Today, I want you to think about how your moods have changed over the past several weeks. Have you noticed an improvement? Are you feeling better about yourself? Better, in general? What we eat certainly affects our mood, but so do our conscious choices. Write down three reasons why your day will go better if you strive to maintain a positive attitude. Today, work toward responding in a positive way to the situations that arise.

WEEK 4 🦋 DAY 3

Today 's Thin Thought: Anything can be done with the right motivation.

Your daily assignments:
- Drink lots of water.
- Bend, stretch, and move upon waking.
- Walk in the morning for at least twenty minutes.
- Keep track of what you put in your mouth.
- Watch your servings/portions.
- Watch your intake of unhealthy fats.
- Move more during the day.
- Choose whole foods over fragmented foods.

Your weekly assignment:
- Weigh yourself.

SETTING THE DAY FOR SUCCESS

If you're like me, you're probably still trying to figure out GI versus GL. It took me a bit to understand it as well, and I've been working with food and weight issues for twenty years! Don't sweat it; just be aware of it because of the tremendous ramifications to your health and *Thin over 40* lifestyle. The Glycemic Index was first created to assist diabetics. The rate of adult-onset diabetes is rising rapidly, and too many people over forty are finding themselves with either full-blown diabetes or becoming prediabetic. Diabetes is a condition where the body can no longer produce the amount of insulin needed to regulate blood sugar. It has long-range health complications, from heart disease to circulation problems.

Research indicates that diabetes and insulin resistance can be caused by the overconsumption of foods with a high Glycemic Index. Type 2 diabetes, the adult-onset type that affects the vast majority of those with diabetes, includes a condition where even though the body produces some insulin, the body does not use it effectively, thus insulin resistance. The net result is the same—too much glucose in the blood. Adult-onset diabetes generally hits people over forty, and is most common in those over fifty-five. Of those with type 2 diabetes, more than 80 percent are overweight. This is why the GI and the GL are important.

What the GI and GL point to, without the need for all of that math, is to be wise about what you eat on a regular basis. This isn't to say that sweets are now totally out of the question. Rather, being a mature individual, given this information about the long-term health ramifications of a steady diet of sweets, you can now make other choices.

And the good news I want to give you is that

eating whole foods can be tasty and wonderful! The more you eat sweets, the more you want them. Conversely, as you begin to decrease the amount of processed, refined sweets, the less you will crave them. It's time to reintroduce that age-old wisdom about the apple. No one ever said a Twinkie a day keeps the doctor away!

SUCCESS IN ACTION

Look over your journal and pick out three highly processed, refined foods you eat on a regular basis. Now, I want you to think about how you can eat those foods differently. For example, if you tend to always have a large helping of ice cream or handful of cookies after dinner, let's look at how you can modify that habit into something healthier.

You could start to replace some of that ice cream with fresh fruit—strawberries, raspberries, or bananas. If you like a handful of cookies after dinner, how about cutting down the number of cookies and including half an apple or a serving of melon? You might even start alternating nights, with one night ice cream and fruit but the next night fruit only. Remember, these are baby steps you are taking. If you say to yourself, "You must not have ice cream ever again!" the first thing you will want to do is eat the whole half gallon. This is about making incremental, positive, lifestyle changes that you can implement for long-term success!

WEEK 4 ❧ DAY 4

Today's Thin Thought: Give yourself permission to eat healthily.

Your daily assignments:
- **Drink lots of water.**

- Bend, stretch, and move upon waking.
- Walk in the morning for at least twenty minutes.
- Keep track of what you put in your mouth.
- Watch your servings/portions.
- Watch your intake of unhealthy fats.
- Move more during the day.
- Choose whole foods over fragmented foods.

SETTING THE DAY FOR SUCCESS

How are you doing with your "no-snack zones?" Have you found it a struggle not to snack during the day? If that's the case, you're not alone, because most people do. Snacking seems to be a way of life. Until now, I didn't want you to snack because of the types of snacks most people eat—high-fat, high-sugar, high-salt foods—and because I wanted you to develop a habit of reaching for your water instead of that candy, cookie, or salty snack.

However, as your metabolism level rises in conjunction with your increased activity level, you may find you need a small snack, an energy perk, in the midmorning or midafternoon. After all, you're burning more calories than you used to. Go ahead and have a snack, if you need one. But the snack must be from whole foods. Choose an apple or orange. A small bran muffin. A handful of almonds. A serving of baby carrots or broccoli. Some soy nuts or dried peas. Remember to continue to drink your water along with your snack. Be satisfied with that small snack, knowing that it will tide you over until you can eat a full meal later.

Make sure to continue to write down your snacks and the amount of calories in them. You should not be eating such large portions that the amount of calories equals a meal.

SUCCESS IN ACTION

When you read you could reintroduce snacks into your day, how did that make you feel? Relieved? Apprehensive? Discouraged that it could only be a "healthy" snack? As we're talking about Food and Mood, what mood do you associate with healthy snacks? Be aware this week of what prompts you to want a snack and which foods you choose. Determine whether it was the food you really wanted or just the distraction of eating.

WEEK 4 🦋 DAY 5

Today's Thin Thought: Variety is the spice of life.

Your daily assignments:
- **Drink lots of water.**
- **Bend, stretch, and move upon waking.**
- **Walk in the morning for at least twenty minutes.**
- **Keep track of what you put in your mouth.**
- **Watch your servings/portions.**
- **Watch your intake of unhealthy fats.**
- **Move more during the day.**
- **Choose a *variety* of whole foods over fragmented foods.**

SETTING THE DAY FOR SUCCESS

As we've looked this week at increasing metabolism by choosing whole foods over fragmented foods, I want you to consider the role variety has in this process. A common aspect of eating disorders—not to mention extreme diets—is the adherence to a short list of "safe" foods. I had one patient who consumed so many carrots, her skin developed an orange tint. The joy of eating foods that stimulate your metabolism is that there are so many of them out there! The *Thin over 40* lifestyle is about the freedom to eat healthy, not the enslavement to a small number of "safe" foods. It's about expanding your choices of good food to eat, not limiting them. Dieting is all about restriction, while *Thin over 40* is about choice.

Now, I know some of you are muttering to yourself, "But what if I choose to eat brownies!" Like many of us, you've probably developed a certain number of comfort foods that you eat consistently. That high-calorie, high-caffeine drink on the way to work. That chocolate doughnut in the morning. That Snickers bar in the afternoon. You probably didn't vary that much.

Now, contrast the *Thin over 40* whole-food approach. You have an entire cornucopia of fruits and vegetables to choose from, all kinds of choices you wouldn't have considered a month ago! Instead of always using white bread on your sandwich, you can choose rye, barley, cracked wheat, sprouted wheat. Instead of always eating beef or chicken for protein, you can try halibut, pork, cod, salmon, even beans.

The only restrictions involved are those you put on yourself by consistently choosing unhealthy ways to fuel your body. That way of eating was restrictive—it kept you lethargic, overweight, unmotivated, and feeling terrible. Do you really want that kind of "freedom" back? I know I don't!

SUCCESS IN ACTION

In the back of this book, you will find a Resource List, where you will find several cookbooks listed.

Your assignment today is to look over that list, go to your local bookstore, and purchase one of them. However, don't be limited to just what's on the list once you get there. If you find a whole-food, fresh-food cookbook with recipes and meal plans that really appeal to you and are in line with what you've been learning, feel free to get that instead! What I want you to do is to begin to expand your horizons by choosing recipes and ingredients you've never tried before. There's a world of culinary possibilities out there waiting for you!

WEEK 4   🦋   DAY 6

Today's Thin Thought: Sometimes your heart's desire is no farther than your own backyard.

Your daily assignments:
- Drink lots of water.
- Bend, stretch, and move upon waking.
- Walk in the morning for at least twenty minutes.
- Keep track of what you put in your mouth.
- Watch your servings/portions.
- Watch your intake of unhealthy fats.
- Move more during the day.
- Choose a variety of whole foods over fragmented foods.

Weekly Assignment:
- Go grocery shopping for next week.

My thanks to Dorothy Gale from *The Wizard of Oz* for today's Thin Thought!

As you look to expand your variety of whole foods, you may find that you need to shop at different stores. This may run counter to your established routine, which is just fine! If today is your Saturday, it's a perfect day to go visit a store you've never been to before (yes, you'll be doing your shopping today instead of Sunday), perhaps one that advertises an especially fresh selection of fruits and vegetables, or fresh fish. Some people think that it's going to be difficult to find the kinds of whole foods they want. However, these foods are available in most communities. But you may have to do a little scouting to find the best sources.

Using your new cookbook, choose a recipe for a dish you've never had before, with ingredients that are new to you. Maybe it's a different type of vegetable or a new herb. Today's the day to experiment! If the weather is nice, and it's the appropriate time of year, get out and explore an area farmers market or outside produce stand. Intentionally buy a fruit or vegetable you haven't tried before. Perhaps it's a different type of apple or one of the imported tropical fruits.

Why go to all this bother? Because I want you to concentrate on the positive choices you are able to make instead of lamenting about the poor eating habits you are committing to discontinue. Again, it's about attitude. It's about Food and Mood. If you feel you're being deprived, you may choose to exhibit a poor attitude. If you embrace this change as a positive, beneficial one, your mood is bound to be better.

SUCCESS IN ACTION
Write down the choice you have made for your new dish. List the ingredients you will need to purchase during your trip out to the various stores in your area. Write down which stores you plan to investigate and include any fresh fruit stands, where applicable. Make sure while you are out to get your

fresh groceries for the next week. Try not to get the majority in one store, but purchase from several. You want to find and support those businesses that will help you in your desire to be *Thin over 40*.

Don't limit yourself just to the produce section. Be aware of what is available in each store's deli or prepared-food section. (Be aware also of how most grocery stores market what they sell, putting candy and snack items near the checkout aisles to take advantage of impulse buying. Once you've made your selections, stand firm and don't be swayed by what's on the rack as you check out!) It's great to know which stores have healthy, whole-food prepared salads and other dishes for times when you're under the gun. These alternatives could save you from feeling the necessity of pulling into a fast-food restaurant if pressed for time.

In addition, your support for these types of products will help ensure that the store continues to provide them and, hopefully, expands their selection of healthy choices. Be a proactive consumer by communicating what types of foods are important to you! Find those stores that recognize and cater to your choices.

WEEK 4   ❦   DAY 7

Today's Thin Thought: To change, you need to be open to possibilities.

Your daily assignments:
- **Drink lots of water.**
- **Bend, stretch, and move upon waking.**
- **Walk in the morning for at least twenty minutes.**
- **Keep track of what you put in your mouth.**
- **Watch your servings/portions.**

- Watch your intake of unhealthy fats.
- Move more during the day.
- Choose a variety of whole foods over frag-
  mented foods.

As you put the finishing touches on Week 4, allow
me to extend my gratitude for your willingness to
continue. I know it takes courage, dedication, and
commitment! I take pride in your courage and add
my own dedication and commitment. These principles work and my desire is for you to keep integrating them into your life. It's astonishing to me how
many people give up on their bodies and their fu-
tures over forty, but you're not one of them! So keep
going! Please know I'm cheering you on!

SETTING THE DAY FOR SUCCESS

If this is your Sunday, it's obviously the weekend.
And weekends are prime time for individuals and
families to enjoy going out to eat at a restaurant. In
Week 2, one of your assignments was to go out to
eat, order what you've always ordered before, but
divide that large restaurant-sized portion into two
meals. As we think about choices, I'd like you to also
consider that you can go to your favorite restaurant
and be proactive about choosing a dish that makes
the most of whole foods. You might also decide to
try some different restaurants to see what choices
they have available. Here are some suggestions, to
give you an idea of how this might work:

- Choose a colorful, flavorful salad for dinner instead of a heavier, fried meal. Use an oil or vinegar
  dressing instead of a creamed selection.
- If you enjoy going to an Italian restaurant, order
  a fresh vegetable antipasto before the meal. This

way, you can order a smaller à la carte selection instead of a full meal.

- Order a baked potato or rice pilaf instead of french fries or mashed potatoes and gravy.
- Forego the chips and salsa at your favorite Mexican restaurant and order fajitas, with their variety of sautéed vegetables. Fajitas also allow you to choose what you put into the tortillas and how many tortillas you eat.
- For dessert, ask for a bowl of fresh fruit or order a piece of fruit pie, and leave the crust, with its high concentration of trans fats. Eat the fruit, not the fat!

Above all, be positive about the possibilities this new way of eating will mean for you. Be alert to how much better you feel during the day. Your food choices really can have an affect on your mood and your attitude each day. Keep an optimistic, positive attitude and allow your food choices to support that decision.

SUCCESS IN ACTION

Your attitude about making these changes is so important. I want you to spend time today concentrating on all of the positive reasons for adopting the *Thin over 40* lifestyle, and specifically for making these whole-food choices.

List your five favorite foods. They can be any kind. Determine which ones you can continue eating as usual. Are there any you should really cut back on? If so, write down your reasons for giving yourself permission to eat less. Frankly, you shouldn't have to eliminate any of your favorite foods altogether. You may just have to save that food for a special, sporadic occasion. As you work toward reducing the amount of high-fat, high-sugar foods you eat, you may find that you become satisfied with a much smaller portion of that food you love so much. I've even had patients who reach a point where that food is no longer appealing to them. Again, it's about freedom. Freedom to choose and not feel chained to certain foods.

HERO OF THE WEEK

As we're talking this week about Food and Mood, there is really only one person I can think of who so completely melds good, healthy food with an incredibly positive, upbeat mood—my friend Graham Kerr. I have had the privilege of his endorsement on other books I have done on healthy eating, and he remains an inspiration to me personally and professionally. His enthusiasm and joy for life overflow in everything he does, including that for which he is most known—cooking! In the Resource List you will find a cookbook of his, *Graham Kerr's Creative Choices Cookbook*. This is a wonderful cookbook that allows the reader to explore the tremendous possibilities of the flavor, taste, and texture of healthy foods. (I encourage you to go to his Web site at www.grahamkerr.com for a full list of books available and information on his latest cooking show.) For being on the forefront of healthy eating, Graham Kerr is my Hero of the Week!

WEEK 5
MAKING THE MOST OF SUPPLEMENTS

WEEK 5 🦋 DAY 1

Today's Thin Thought: You don't get everything you need from the food you eat.

I am so proud of you! Here we are, beginning our fifth week of the *Thin over 40* Plan. This week we are going to be taking a look at the role of nutritional supplements and proper adrenal and thyroid functioning. For those of us over forty, maintaining a healthy weight and energy level can be more complicated than keeping your food intake down to a set number of calories per day. Over forty, we need to be strategic not only about what nutrients we get from food, but also about ways we can support our bodies through nutritional supplementation. The research is exciting and encouraging!

Your daily assignments:
- **Drink lots of water.** Remember, you're working toward eight to ten cups per day.
- **Bend, stretch, and move upon waking.** Don't skimp on this time!
- **Walk in the morning for at least twenty-five minutes.** You're building on your time every two weeks. Research shows that walking even one mile per day can keep you from a one to three pound yearly weight gain!

- **Keep track of what you put in your mouth.** Be accountable to yourself by writing it down.
- **Watch your servings/portions.** Learn to enjoy your food, not merely inhale it.
- **Watch your intake of unhealthy fats.** Keep reading the back of those boxes!
- **Move more during the day.** Carve out time for your health every day. It benefits you and those around you.
- **Choose a variety whole foods over fragmented foods.** Remember to look for variety and keep adding to your list of personal favorites.

SETTING THE DAY FOR SUCCESS

The Key Concept for this week is the role of the Adrenals. Your adrenal system and your thyroid work together to regulate your body's production of hormones. (We'll deal more with hormones in Week 8.) If your adrenals are overworked or stressed, the thyroid automatically turns the metabolic rate down in order to "calm" the system. This reduction in metabolic rate means weight gain. It is important, therefore, to identify ways your adrenal system can be stressed.

According to Dr. Joseph Mercola, an osteopathic physician and founder of one of the most visited health Web sites (www.mercola.com), there are a variety of causes for adrenal stress.[1] Basically, what puts stress on the body, puts stress on the adrenals—excessive anger and worry, feeling guilty, overworking, not getting enough sleep, exposure to toxins, hypoglycemia, nutritional deficiencies, trauma, and injury.

1. Mercola, Joseph, http://www.mercola.com/2000/aug/27/adrenals.htm.

Another important stressor is, frankly, the way we eat. When we feed our body a steady diet of caffeine and sugar, we rob it of the nutrients needed to do its job. Not only do we rob it by what we do eat, we rob it by what we don't eat. The body was meant to obtain a majority of its calories through fresh fruits and vegetables, lean meats, and whole grains. Our mass-produced, highly processed, chemically saturated foods stress out our systems and wreck havoc with their ability to function optimally. The good news is that a return to healthier eating and the use of nutritional supplements can assist the body and reduce stress to our adrenal system.

SUCCESS IN ACTION

Look over the following list from Dr. Mercola and write down any that are present in your own life. Be honest about how much of a role these play in a typical day.

Common Causes of Adrenal Stress[2]

- Anger
- Fear
- Worry/anxiety
- Depression
- Guilt
- Overwork/physical or mental strain
- Excessive exercise
- Sleep deprivation
- Light-cycle disturbance
- Going to sleep late
- Surgery
- Trauma/injury
- Chronic inflammation
- Chronic infection

2. Ibid, page 4.

- Chronic pain
- Temperature extremes
- Toxic exposure
- Malabsorption
- Maldigestion
- Chronic illness
- Chronic severe allergies
- Hypoglycemia
- Nutritional deficiencies

Your body works very hard each and every day to cope with the ups and downs of life. You can see from the list the number and variety of factors that can have a negative impact and drain on your adrenal health. The more stress you're under, the more important it is to eat healthy to support your body nutritionally. For some of us, this list represents far too many factors in our daily lives. What is true for you? Can you understand how vital it is to consider the food you eat every day as a way to strengthen, repair, and maintain your physical systems? If you don't, that body of yours will break down. An aging body needs to be built up!

WEEK 5 🦋 DAY 2

Today's Thin Thought: How you live your life affects how your body reacts and responds.

Your daily assignments:
- **Drink lots of water.**
- **Bend, stretch, and move upon waking.**
- **Walk in the morning for at least twenty-five minutes.**
- **Keep track of what you put in your mouth.**
- **Watch your servings/portions.**
- **Watch your intake of unhealthy fats.**
- **Move more during the day.**

- Choose a variety of whole foods over fragmented foods.
- Take a good multivitamin/multimineral.

SETTING THE DAY FOR SUCCESS

How you live your life affects how your body is able to respond and react. The more stress you put on it, the less able it is to respond positively. When adrenals are maxed, it affects the thyroid. Listen to this quote from the husband-and-wife team of Richard L. and Karilee Halo Shames in *Thyroid Power: 10 Steps to Total Health*:

> Our country is in the grip of yet another energy crisis. Both men and women are working harder, demanding more of themselves, and are pressured to get more done in less time. With the increased pace of life and the increased chemical contamination of our air, food, and water, people are more than simply work exhausted or stressed out. Many are actually developing a chronic, low-energy illness.
>
> One of the most common places for this energy illness to strike is the thyroid gland. . . . When this gland is hampered by illness, causing reduced production of thyroid hormone, every bodily function is diminished."[3]

We are burning our bodies out by the pace we adopt and the amount of stress we put on ourselves. The aging process can be stressful enough! It's time

3. Shames, Richard L., M.D., and Karilee Halo Shames, R.N., Ph.D. *Thyroid Power: 10 Steps to Total Health*. New York: First Quill/HarperResource, 2002, page 6.

to support our bodies as we age, instead of living a life that wears us down even faster! Again, from the Shames, ". . . the increasingly rapid pace of life may leave little time for immune-restoring activities such as aerobic exercise, muscle building, or slow stretching."[4] Aerobic exercise (your walking), muscle building (your work with weights), and slow stretching (your morning routine)! This should fortify your resolve to continue in your *Thin over 40* commitment!

There is more you can do to support your body. Today, if you are not doing so already, I want you to start taking a good multi-vitamin, multi-mineral supplement. Now, don't turn your nose up at this! It used to be that even the idea of taking vitamins for health was considered kooky or "alternative." Supplements were thought to be of little use or value compared to traditional Western medicine. Now, even the American Medical Association has come out with a recommendation that all adults take a daily multivitamin, multimineral supplement.

Not all multis are the same, however. Look for a supplement that has a broad base of vitamins and minerals, including trace elements. A comprehensive supplement formula has the ingredients necessary for the body to take advantage of each one of the supplements. For example, most people have heard of the benefits of taking a calcium supplement, especially in later life. But calcium needs phosphorous for the body to assimilate it properly. Taking one without the other reduces the benefit.

Here are the components to look for in a multi-formula: vitamin A, vitamin B_6, vitamin B_{12}, vitamin C, vitamin D, vitamin E, thiamin, riboflavin, niacin, folic acid, biotin, pantothenic acid, calcium, phospho-

4. Ibid, page 13.

rous, iodine, magnesium, zinc, selenium, copper, manganese, chromium, molybdenum, and potassium. (For an example of amounts of each of these, go to my Web site at www.aplaceofhope.com and go to the online store, Nutritional Supplements. You can look up the specific information on the multiformula we use at The Center, called Multi/Mineral Plus.)

In addition, you need a formula that your body can actually use. The terms you want to look for on the label are "optimal absorption" and "bioavailability." Basically, this means that your body is actually able to use and absorb the product. Avoid those with a high level of inorganic minerals like oyster shell, dolomite, calcium carbonate, or magnesium oxide. These are not from plant/organic sources and are too hard for the body to digest. If you have any trouble digesting a multi, try switching to a type that you take in doses several times a day. Some people find that iron can upset their stomach or cause constipation, so if necessary, switch to a formula without iron.

SUCCESS IN ACTION

Think about the idea of taking a pill (multi-formula) for the rest of your life. Does it make you feel old? Do you resent the idea that you'll be "tied down" taking this pill? If you have been taking a vitamin/mineral supplement, how's it going? Are you consistent? Are there days you take it and days you don't? Do you have the same feeling about any medications you are currently taking? Are you as diligent about your vitamins as you are about your medications? If not, why not?

If you encounter a roadblock to taking your vitamins, find a way around it! Because this is so important, I want you to be successful! Find a logical place to put the vitamin bottle, where you will remember

to access it each and every day. If you need to take
your vitamins during the day, keep a small container
at work, in your briefcase or purse (small plastic film
canisters work great!).

WEEK 5   🦋   DAY 3

*Today's Thin Thought: Your path in the
morning sets your course for the day.*

Your daily assignments:
- Drink lots of water.
- Bend, stretch, and move upon waking.
- Walk in the morning for at least twenty-
  five minutes.
- Keep track of what you put in your mouth.
- Watch your servings/portions.
- Watch your intake of unhealthy fats.
- Move more during the day.
- Choose a variety of whole foods over frag-
  mented foods.
- Take a good multivitamin/multimineral.

Your weekly assignment:
- Weigh yourself.

SETTING THE DAY FOR SUCCESS

With your current routine of moving your body
and reviving your metabolism in the morning, you're
already setting a great course for the day. I'd like
you to consider another excellent way to start your
morning off right. This becomes especially important
after your morning walk. Right after you've exer-
cised, your body needs protein in amino acids to replenish and repair itself. Most typical breakfast foods
are extremely high in carbohydrates in relationship

to protein. Add to that our fast-paced world and breakfast can become a danish on the run or a bowl of cereal gulped down during a quick read of the Sports section. We really need better than that. My recommendation is to invest in a good-quality, well-balanced protein drink to get your morning started off right. These drinks contain a good mix of proteins, carbohydrates, vitamins, and minerals, while remaining low in calories. They can be made quickly and are very potable.

I first became a fan of protein drinks through our work with eating disorder clients. So often, an eating disorder depletes the body's store of nutrients and decimates the digestive system. We needed to find a product that our clients could use in the morning that was easy to digest and tolerate, with highly absorbable nutrients and without any of the common food allergy "trigger" ingredients, such as dairy, egg, wheat, or gluten.

After many years of seeing how successful this was for our eating-disorder clients, I realized it could be good for me, too! In fact, it can also be great for those wanting to manage hypertension, metabolic syndrome, estrogen imbalance, and weight. We use UltraMeal by Metagenics, but there are other good brands on the market. When looking for a powdered protein drink (and you don't' have to have it in the morning, by the way), pay careful attention to the ingredient list. Avoid any products that tout themselves solely for weight reduction. Ironically, one of the most popular shakes for weight loss lists numerous types of sugar right on the label. (It won't say sugar, of course, but look for any ingredient that ends in "ose," such as fructose, lactose, or sucrose. All of these are sugars. Anytime you see "ose," think sugar.)

You're looking for a product that closely mirrors a good multimineral vitamin formula—and still tastes good! Ask for a sample when you're able. Try blending it with milk or water and a little ice. You can also blend in a serving of fresh fruit to make a smoothie. Starting your morning with a protein/supplement mix is a great way to give your body what it needs to meet the demands of the morning, as well as establish a healthy glucose level from the start.

SUCCESS IN ACTION

Mornings used to be a time to prepare for the day. With as hectic as life can be over forty, many people greet the morning with the panicked thought that they are already behind! This adds untold stress and provides a built-in excuse for neglecting a nutritious start to the day in favor of a quick caffeine- or fat-laden infusion in the mad dash to work.

I'd like you to spend some time with your journal today, writing about a typical morning. How has it changed since you began *Thin over 40*? Contrast how your day progresses when you've had a "good" morning as compared to a "bad" morning. How do you feel physically? Emotionally? How is your attitude toward yourself and others? Day after day of unrelenting pressure and stress isn't good for your attitude—or your adrenals!

WEEK 5   🦋   DAY 4

Today's Thin Thought: Not all fats are evil.

Your daily assignments:
- Drink lots of water.
- Bend, stretch, and move upon waking.
- Walk in the morning for at least twenty-five minutes.

- Keep track of what you put in your mouth.
- Watch your servings/portions.
- Watch your intake of unhealthy fats.
- Move more during the day.
- Choose a variety of whole foods over fragmented foods.
- Take a good multivitamin/multimineral.

SETTING THE DAY FOR SUCCESS

Today we're going to talk about fats. You've already become aware of the negative consequences of bad fats in your diet—the saturated fats and trans fats. As we look at the benefits of nutritional supplementation this week, I'd like you to consider a fat that is actually good for you. It's the omega-3 fats found in cold-water-fish oil. These are also known as EPA (Eicosapentaenoic acid) and DHA (Docosahexaenoic acid). Together, these essential fatty acids do a world of good. They give you a healthy balance of triglycerides. They support proper nervous system function, along with cardiovascular health and immune system function. In fact, these fats are important to every hormone system and all new cell production. (Recommended doses are 300 to 500 mg for EPA and 250 to 400 mgs of DHA per day.)

Why not just eat the fish? Go ahead and eat fish, but be aware that some types of fish, such as tuna, shark, and swordfish, can have high levels of heavy metals. Taking an EPA/DHA supplement is a great way to increase the amount of omega-3 in your diet, especially for those who don't necessarily like fish. Omega-3 fats are also found in flaxseed, safflower oil, and walnuts. One of the common complaints of taking fish oil is burping up the taste. Freezing the capsules can reduce this unpleasant side effect.

SUCCESS IN ACTION

I want you to start a supplement checklist today. As you read about different options during this week, write down those that especially appeal to you, so you can head out this weekend and do some supplement sleuthing—determining where you can obtain these products. It may mean calling on the phone, looking on the Internet, or visiting a local supplement store. All of the supplements talked about during this week are also available online through www.thinover40.com.

WEEK 5 🦋 DAY 5

Today's Thin Thought: Big improvements can come from tiny components.

Your daily assignments:
- **Drink lots of water.**
- **Bend, stretch, and move upon waking.**
- **Walk in the morning for at least twenty-five minutes.**
- **Keep track of what you put in your mouth.**
- **Watch your servings/portions.**
- **Watch your intake of unhealthy fats.**
- **Move more during the day.**
- **Choose a variety of whole foods over fragmented foods.**
- **Take a good multivitamin/multimineral.**

SETTING THE DAY FOR SUCCESS

Today I want to talk about two nutritional supplements that specifically help the functioning of the mitochondria. Now, you may not have heard that word since high-school science! It's very easy to overlook these cellular dynamos. Though tiny, they have a big job to do in the body. Mitochondria in cells act as little furnaces where fat is burned. They cannot leave the cell and go to where the fat is, so the fat must come to them. Therein lies the benefit of the two supplements I want to introduce to you today, L-Carnitine and Coenzyme Q10.

L-Carnitine is an amino acid required for the breakdown of fats into energy. It acts as a carrier, transporting fats to the mitochondria, where they can be burned as fuel. The easier fat is burned, the more efficient your physical activity becomes. The more fat burned as fuel, the less stored on your body. The more fat burned, the lower your cholesterol drops. (Recommended dose is 500 mg per day.)

Coenzyme Q10 (ubiquinone) also supports energy production in the mitochondria, thus increasing your metabolism. In addition, studies have shown it to have antioxidant properties, removing cancer-causing free radicals from your system and promoting cardiac muscle health. As you strive to live a *Thin over 40* lifestyle, it makes sense to utilize supplements that will assist you in that goal. As you increase your physical activity, your body will want to burn off excess fat to fuel that increase. These supplements can help your body in that goal! (Recommended dose is 30-60 mg per day.)

SUCCESS IN ACTION

Today, I want you to get in front of a mirror and really look at your body. Note the areas where excess fat has been stored—your upper arms, your stomach, around the shoulder blades, inside your thighs, under your chin. Now, imagine how you will look as those areas are reduced and replaced with healthy muscle tissue. That's the *Thin over 40* you, worth all of this education and effort. You are worth it! Write

down that affirmation today in your journal—"I am
worth it!" in large, bold letters—reiterating your
commitment.

WEEK 5   🦋   DAY 6

*Today's Thin Thought: A new direction requires
a new perspective.*

Your daily assignments:
- Drink lots of water.
- Bend, stretch, and move upon waking.
- Walk in the morning for at least twenty-
  five minutes.
- Keep track of what you put in your mouth.
- Watch your servings/portions.
- Watch your intake of unhealthy fats.
- Move more during the day.
- Choose a variety of whole foods over frag-
  mented foods.
- Take a good multivitamin/multimineral.

SETTING THE DAY FOR SUCCESS

Good morning! As we near the end of Week 5, I
want us to look at two more major nutritional supplements today. The first is CLA (conjugated linoleic
acid). CLA has been shown to reduce body fat without a corresponding loss of lean muscle mass. Remember, the more lean muscle we have, the higher
our metabolic rate, even when resting. Since 1999,
this supplement has been used and studied for its
effect on the reduction of body fat in animals and
people. (Recommended dose is 3.4 grams or above.)
Please be aware that some CLA supplements come
with a slow-releasing caffeine component called
guarana.

The other supplement I'd like to bring to your attention today is probably one you're already familiar with. It's the dual supplement glucosamine (glucosamine hydrochloride) and chondroitin (chondroitin sulfate). Glucosamine helps with the production of cartilage and connective tissue. Chondroitin protects existing cartilage and also helps to form new cartilage. Together, they are wonderful for joint health and repair.

As we age, one of the areas where many people experience pain and inflammation is in their joints. It hurts to move, reducing a desire for physical activity in response. By taking a glucosamine/chondroitin supplement, you are safeguarding the cartilage you have and giving your body what it needs to rebuild and repair damaged joints. From elbows to knees, from shoulders to hips to ankles, in order to live an active *Thin over 40* life, you need to be proactive in cushioning the wear and tear on your joints. This is a popular dietary supplement sold in most grocery stores and nutrition outlets. (Recommended dose is 4500 mg of glucosamine and 3600 mg of chondroitin.)

SUCCESS IN ACTION

Today I want you to complete your supplement list in your journal and use that as a guide to pick up the ones that especially appeal to you. If all of them do, go ahead and purchase them! If you are a bit wary and want to try just a few at a time to see how it goes, I recommend—besides the multivitamin/multimineral—the omega-3 essential fatty acids and the glucosamine/chondroitin. Use these products over the following weeks of *Thin over 40*, making sure to journal any changes you observe to your energy, mood, and physical flexibility. As you notice positive changes, be open to adding other of the supplements explained during this week.

For those of you concerned about the cost of these supplements, consider the money you have spent in the past on things that no longer matter to you. What you spend your money on shows what you value. Isn't it time you valued yourself and your health?

WEEK 5   🌿   DAY 7

Today's Thin Thought: If drawing from a dry well, don't be surprised when you come up empty.

Your daily assignments:
- **Drink lots of water.**
- **Bend, stretch, and move upon waking.**
- **Walk in the morning for at least twenty-five minutes.**
- **Keep track of what you put in your mouth.**
- **Watch your servings/portions.**
- **Watch your intake of unhealthy fats.**
- **Move more during the day.**
- **Choose a variety of whole foods over fragmented foods.**
- **Take a good multivitamin/multimineral.**

Weekly Assignment:
- **Go grocery shopping for next week.**

SETTING THE DAY FOR SUCCESS

Well, you've had a lot to think about this week. For some of you, this whole concept of nutritional supplements might still seem like so much smoke and mirrors. I have experienced too much in my own life and seen too much in the lives of others where supplements are concerned, to ever entertain this thought. When the body is supported with the nutrients it needs, amazing progress is possible. When the body is not supported, either through diet, lifestyle, or both, damage occurs that can have long-range effects, both physical and psychological.

Think about it like building a retaining wall. You can use cheap materials, unsupported, and the wall will probably look just fine at first. But over time, with the effects of wind and rain and the natural shifting of the earth behind that wall, the foundation becomes undermined. It will begin to bulge in all the wrong places. Pieces of it may even drop off. The quality of the materials and the construction will invariably begin to show over time. What looked great when it was young now shows its age and more. In order for the wall to function properly again, it needs to be shored up and parts that are damaged replaced.

Poor eating habits don't show their effects immediately. It takes time to really highlight the deficiencies. Time acts as a corrosive agent all by itself. But when you add in the stress of life, deterioration can accelerate. This double onslaught against your body—years of unhealthy eating and stress—is what causes many people to experience significant physical problems over forty. If that is the case with you, your decision to commit to *Thin over 40* is allowing you to repair the damage done. Your daily assignments are, brick by brick, strengthening you to take advantage of all life has to offer over forty. Please be patient—the more damage that has been done to your wall, the longer it will take to rebuild. But be assured that every positive step has tremendous benefit.

For those of you with a particular interest in the adrenals and thyroid system, I heartily recommend two books for you to consider for further study. The first has already been mentioned, *Thyroid Power* by the Shames. The second is *Adrenal Fatigue: The 21st Century Stress Syndrome* by James L. Wilson, N.D., D.C., Ph.D. See the Resource List at the back of this book for more information.

SUCCESS IN ACTION

In your journal, I want you to draw a large square—this is your "wall." Now, divide the wall up into sixteen "bricks"—using 4 x 4 lines. In each brick, I want you to put something positive you are doing. You can already fill up at least ten: This book, water, stretching, walking, tracking food, tracking portions, less bad fats, more movement, whole foods, multis. Now, in the remaining six squares, write down things you have added yourself as you've worked through the book or specific supplements you have decided to take.

Now, look at your full wall. A continued commitment to each of the squares is going to represent a strong, supported physical and psychological life from this day forward!

HERO OF THE WEEK

In years past, the traditional medical community has been less than supportive of individuals who sought to deal with aging and a variety of health concerns through the use of nutritional supplements. Instead, the answer was increasingly pharmaceutical, with more and more people on more and more medications. Thankfully, this mind-set is beginning to shift. On the leading edge of this shift has been my friend Dr. Maurice Stephens, who now works with us at The Center. Trained as a medical doctor, he has dedicated his knowledge and expertise to understanding the role of nutrition and lifestyle in assisting with the prevention and mitigation of health concerns. Whenever possible, Dr. Stephens advocates for commonsense, practical changes to enhance life and functioning. His infectious good humor and sincere depth of caring are truly remarkable! For his steadfast belief in the ability of the body to heal and accomplish amazing results, Dr. Maurice Stephens is my Hero of the Week!

WEEK 6
MAKING THE MOST OF YOUR BRAIN POWER

WEEK 6 🦋 DAY 1

Today's Thin Thought: Understanding is power.

Welcome to Week 6 of *Thin Over 40*! This week marks the halfway point in your journey to lifelong health and vitality. You've been staying with your commitment for a month and a half—congratulations! There's great information still ahead. This week, we will be looking at how our brains function and how that functioning affects our body and our body's ability to maintain a healthy weight.

Your daily assignments:
- **Drink lots of water.** Now is not the time to relax your focus on this. Continue to be proactive by keeping water with you at all times.
- **Bend, stretch, and use your weights upon waking.** You should be working into a routine that makes sense for you and your physical condition. Keep at it!
- **Walk in the morning for at least twenty-five minutes.** Look forward to this time, just for you!
- **Keep track of what you put in your mouth.** Keep track and make intentional, healthy choices.
- **Watch your servings/portions.** When in doubt, measure it out!

- **Watch your intake of unhealthy fats.** Be aware of hidden sources in processed foods.
- **Move more during the day.** All through the day and in the evening after dinner.
- **Choose a variety of whole foods over fragmented foods.** Learn to enjoy flavor, texture, and crunch over sweet and salty.
- **Enhance your diet with nutritional supplements.** Ask questions, find answers, and give them a try.
- **Take a good multivitamin/multimineral.**

SETTING THE DAY FOR SUCCESS

This week, we'll examine the effects of four key brain chemicals, or neurotransmitters, on maximizing your *Thin over 40* success. Those brain chemicals are: GABA, endorphins, dopamine, and serotonin. The Key Concept for Week 6, therefore, is Brain Power. For many of you, this is going to be new information. You have a basic understanding of how your body works but you've probably relied on doctors to explain any definable injury or illness. After sharing your concern or complaint, you came away with a prescription or an admonition not to do again whatever caused the problem in the first place. I venture to say that few of you have had an in-depth discussion with your physician about the effects of neurotransmitters; if you've even heard the term, it was probably in the context of a prescription for one of the antidepressant medications such as Prozac, Paxil, Zoloft, or Effexor, which promote increased serotonin levels.

These brain chemicals each have a specific function in regulating how you respond to pleasure, stress, and pain. GABA (gamma-aminobutyric acid) is actually an amino acid that acts as a neurotransmitter, which is a fancy way of saying it facilitates communication between brain cells. Neurotransmitters allow brains cells to "talk" to each other.

GABA also stimulates that part of the brain that produces HGH (human growth hormone). HGH helps the body create lean muscle mass and lose fat. As we age, our bodies reduce production of HGH, so GABA is important in counteracting this effect. GABA also acts as an inhibitor of pain, fear, and attention, allowing the body to relax and sleep. Its counterpart, glutamate, acts as an excitant. Or, as Richard A. Morrisett, associate professor of pharmacology at The University of Texas at Austin, puts it, "Glutamate is the accelerator pedal and GABA is the brake pedal. GABA essentially shuts the brain off."[1]

SUCCESS IN ACTION

Today I'd like you to think about the role relaxation plays in your day-to-day life. The faster and faster you accelerate during your day—through your activities, your thoughts, your reactions—the more it takes to "brake" at the end of the day, to relax and rest. To continue the automobile analogy, take a page in your journal and write three headings: "Activities," "Accelerate," and "Decelerate." Beginning in the morning, consider each of your daily activities and indicate whether they tend to "speed you up" or "slow you down." Are you constantly revving down the road of your day, unable to slow down and relax at the end? Do you hit the day already in

1. As quoted in "Neurosteroids: the missing link?" by A. Leslie Morrow, Ph.D. Public Release date: 12/13/1999. http:// www.eurekalert.org/pub_releases/1999-12/ACER-Ntml-131299.php.

second gear? Are your brake pads shot from trying to slow down too much, too fast?

I want you to consciously think about your internal "speed." The more anxious, tense, and excited you are, the more glutamate you produce, requiring greater amounts of GABA to slow you down. Insufficient amounts can lead to anxious, runaway thoughts and a reduction in the kind of deep, restful sleep needed to restock for the next day. (We'll expand more on this concept next week.) Be aware of how your activities and thoughts today affect your internal speed.

WEEK 6 ❦ DAY 2

Today's Thin Thought: Don't worry—relax.

Your daily assignments:
- **Drink lots of water.**
- **Bend, stretch, and move upon waking.**
- **Walk in the morning for at least twenty-five minutes.**
- **Keep track of what you put in your mouth.**
- **Watch your servings/portions.**
- **Watch your intake of unhealthy fats.**
- **Move more during the day.**
- **Choose a variety of whole foods over fragmented foods.**
- **Take a good multivitamin/multimineral.**
- **Enhance your diet with nutritional supplements.**

SETTING THE DAY FOR SUCCESS

Today's Thin Thought is a very simple direction that is extremely complicated to accomplish. Our brains are prepared to produce the chemical we need to accomplish this, but our minds interfere with its ability to do so. With the stress of life after forty, it can be difficult to stop at the end of the day—let alone during the day—and just relax. We're worried about what we didn't get done, whether what we did get done is good enough, what surprises tomorrow might bring, and how we'll have the strength to do it all over again. Anxiety, stress, and tension eat at our ability to lay down our burdens and experience peace.

One of the ways some people have found to achieve a state of relaxation is through the consumption of alcohol. Alcohol in moderation does have certain health benefits. For example, studies have shown that red wine contains an antioxidant, and antioxidants have been shown to protect the body from damage on the cellular level. However, a recent study in the *Journal of Agricultural and Food Chemistry* indicated that the cocoa in hot chocolate has a higher amount of antioxidants than red wine or green tea— twice as high, in fact, as in red wine and two to three times higher than green tea. This certainly offers a delicious alternative for those who don't want to drink alcohol or shouldn't because of a family history of alcoholism.

Another positive link was discovered between alcohol consumption and GABA production. If we think of GABA as the brain's "brake," alcohol increases the amount of "brake fluid" available. In essence, alcohol affects the body by enhancing the inhibiting or relaxing effects of GABA. For those who are able, alcohol in moderation can indeed be a relaxant. But some people may find it difficult to maintain moderate consumption, wreaking havoc on their health and their weight. Fortunately, there are other ways to increase your store of GABA in order to achieve a relaxed, peaceful state. Many of my clients benefit from taking amino acids, the building blocks needed for GABA, and other neurotransmitters talked about during this week. This is especially true of those whose digestive systems have been compromised by an eating disorder or disordered eating, making it difficult for their bodies to properly break down the protein they eat into its component amino acids. For them it is important to find a highly digestible additional source of amino acids. If you find you are having recurring, chronic challenges with energy levels, concentration, clarity of thought, or heightened anxiety, I encourage you to speak to a health care professional about supplementing your diet with an amino acid formula.

SUCCESS IN ACTION

Today I want you to evaluate your alcohol use. How often do you consume alcohol during the week? How much do you consume? Has a family member or friend ever expressed concern over your alcohol consumption? Do you feel like you need a drink in the evening in order to relax? Have you ever fallen asleep after drinking prior to retiring to bed? Do you usually consume alcohol with your meal? Do you drink after your meal as well?

If you do not consume alcohol, consider what you do use to relax at the end of the day. Do you find you are unable to sleep without these things? Make a list of what you use to unwind at the end of the day. There are a variety of wonderful alternatives to alcohol or sleeping pills. Moderate exercise or sexual interaction in the evening is a great way to bring about a state of relaxation. (We'll talk about others next week.)

For those of you who do regularly consume alco-

hol, especially to relax, I'd like you also to consider
the amount of calories involved in this habit. Alcohol
is treated in the body like pure sugar. It also acts
as a depressant, slowing down your metabolism. By
drinking in the evening, you may be relaxing but
you are also adding on calories at the end of your
day, when they're most quickly stored as fat. These
calories must be factored into your weight goals.

WEEK 6 ❧ DAY 3

*Today's Thin Thought: Exercise can be the high
point of your day.*

Your daily assignments:
  • **Drink lots of water.**
  • **Bend, stretch, and move upon waking.**
  • **Walk in the morning for at least twenty-
    five minutes.**
  • **Keep track of what you put in your mouth.**
  • **Watch your servings/portions.**
  • **Watch your intake of unhealthy fats.**
  • **Move more during the day.**
  • **Choose a variety of whole foods over frag-
    mented foods.**
  • **Take a good multivitamin/multimineral.**
  • **Enhance your diet with nutritional supple-
    ments.**

Your weekly assignment:
  • **Weigh yourself.**

SETTING THE DAY FOR SUCCESS

Today I'd like to talk about another of our key
brain chemicals, endorphins. Endorphins are neurotransmitters that reduce the amount of pain we feel.

Endorphins have been called the body's natural opiates. They may be familiar to you, in reference to exercise, or the "runner's high." These natural pain-killers are produced through prolonged, sustained exercise. They produce not only a reduction in pain sensation but also increased feelings of euphoria, a reduction in appetite, and the release of sex hormones. Along with exercise, endorphins are released through a hearty laugh, stressful situations, and sexual activity.

As you look for ways to relax and experience joy in life, don't overlook what you can do for yourself through your own endorphins. When you exercise for a sustained period of time, your body responds to this stress with the release of endorphins. You may not be a runner, but you can still experience a feeling of well-being through exercise. Walking or exercising to music and swimming are also excellent ways to trigger endorphin production. Your objective is not to elicit pain but rather put just the right amount of stress on your body. You're looking for well-being, not stiff, sore muscles.

If you find that you've overdone on your exercise, however, you can still stimulate endorphins through massage. If you have never experienced a therapeutic or deep-muscle massage, I encourage you to do so! Working your muscles in this way will cause your body to release endorphins and allow for increased relaxation. (Be aware that deep-tissue massages, while wonderful, can produce slight headaches or nausea as the body deals with the toxins released through the massage process. This is not a reason to avoid massages, but rather, be wise and make sure to drink lots of water to help flush your system of these toxins.)

SUCCESS IN ACTION

This week, as you are stretching and walking in the morning, I'd like you to add soothing music to your experience, if you haven't done so already. Find a station on the radio you like, or bring along a CD player. It makes no difference what kind of music, as long as it is pleasurable to you. See if you can incorporate the rhythm of the music into your activity, whether it's stretching or walking. You're looking to achieve a state of relaxation, even in the midst of physical exercise. This is the peaceful, contented feeling from your own endorphins!

As a bonus, consider making an appointment for a relaxation massage. If you live in a part of the country where these services are not available (or you do not feel comfortable with the service providers in your area), ask your spouse or a friend to gently massage the muscles in your face, scalp, neck, and back. These are the areas where many of us center our stress reactions. If you're able, consider incorporating a healthful massage on a regular basis. Go ahead and look in the phone book right now and see what might be available where you live. Investigate the services and, if comfortable, make an appointment today!

WEEK 6 🦋 DAY 4

Today's Thin Thought: Appreciate the joys of sex.

Your daily assignments:
- **Drink lots of water.**
- **Bend, stretch, and move upon waking.**
- **Walk in the morning for at least twenty-five minutes.**
- **Keep track of what you put in your mouth.**

- Watch your servings/portions.
- Watch your intake of unhealthy fats.
- Move more during the day.
- Choose a variety of whole foods over fragmented foods.
- Take a good multivitamin/multimineral.
- Enhance your diet with nutritional supplements.

SETTING THE DAY FOR SUCCESS

Today we're going to talk about sex. One of the main ways to experience the euphoria of endorphin release is through sexual stimulation and activity. In addition, sexual arousal promotes the production of HGH. Quite simply, sex can be physically very beneficial. There is a myth that those over forty have a diminished ability to enjoy sex, that really great sex is reserved for your twenties. I believe this misconception has come about because of the statistical drop-off in sexual activity as you age. This can happen for a variety of reasons—illness, injury, emotional difficulties inhibiting sexual intimacy, loss of physical vitality and stamina. Chronic fatigue can also make sex seem unappealing. Most of these conditions can be addressed medically or psychologically, allowing for a return of sexual function.

As you continue through *Thin over 40*, as your energy and stamina increase, you may find that your interest in sex increases also. It works the other way too: maintaining a consistent pattern of sexual activity enhances your quality of life and can help motivate you to continue positive, healthful changes!

Many women I've worked with have expressed the feeling of being sexually unattractive because of their weight. Seeing themselves as unattractive or unlovable, they shut down their sexual feelings and isolate themselves. As you learn to nurture and appreciate your body, you should begin to see yourself again as an attractive, sexual person. You don't need to achieve physical "perfection" before enjoying sexual intimacy!

SUCCESS IN ACTION

The benefits of intimacy are so great that I want everyone who is able to experience them. If your sex life is not what you would like it to be, I encourage you to consult with a medical or counseling professional and investigate whether there is a physical or emotional reason for the difficulties you are experiencing.

Perhaps you feel that your best years, sexually, are behind you. You may be between relationships. In your journal, I'd like you to be honest and record your feelings about yourself and sex. What do you like about it? What don't you like about it? What things do you want to change? How would these changes increase your pleasure in sex? Your frequency of sex? If you are not sexually active, does this change how you view yourself? In what ways?

Now, I understand that some of you reading this book have made a decision to be celibate. In no way do I want to dissuade you from that decision. In your journal instead, articulate your commitment to remain celibate and note other ways you can incorporate physical fulfillment and enjoyment in your life.

WEEK 6   ❦   DAY 5

Today's Thin Thought: Being in the mood can be more than a state of mind.

Your daily assignments:
- **Drink lots of water.**

- Bend, stretch, and move upon waking.
- Walk in the morning for at least twenty-five minutes.
- Keep track of what you put in your mouth.
- Watch your servings/portions.
- Watch your intake of unhealthy fats.
- Move more during the day.
- Choose a variety of whole foods over fragmented foods.
- Take a good multivitamin/multimineral.
- Enhance your diet with nutritional supplements.

SETTING THE DAY FOR SUCCESS

I'd like to continue our discussion of brain chemicals by introducing another—dopamine—that contributes to healthy sexual drive. Dopamine also increases learning and memory, and helps you be more alert. Dopamine is made from the amino acid tyrosine. Tyrosine can be found in dairy products, meats, fish, wheat, oats, and other protein-containing foods. A healthy, well-rounded diet generally provides the necessary supply of tyrosine, but some people may benefit from supplementation. There are some psychiatric disorders, such as schizophrenia, as well as Parkinson's disease, that have been linked to a dopamine imbalance.

The release of dopamine can be triggered by certain foods. Dopamine does not appear to increase the pleasure of the actual food when eaten, but it is released when a person sees, smells, or tastes something they consider enjoyable. No wonder the food is pleasurable! You feel better and become more alert.

This cued response is based upon what each person considers enjoyable. I might love a certain type of food you can't stand. Seeing, smelling, or tasting that food would release a dopamine response in me but not in you. Sometimes, the cued response comes from an experience tied to food, such as cotton candy at the fair, or popcorn at the movies. We've basically told our brains which foods to respond to. What would happen if we reconditioned our brain to enjoy other types of food?

SUCCESS IN ACTION

In your journal today, I want you to think back to some foods you associate with good times and enjoyment. These can be from your childhood to the present. How do those foods make you feel? Do you notice any patterns among the types of foods you put down? Are they sweet? Salty? Do they include fruits and vegetables? Many times, our comfort foods do not consist of broccoli and barley. But could they? Over the last six weeks, have you come to appreciate and enjoy new and healthier foods? Write down some of your new favorites.

Today, as you eat, make sure to savor the flavor of your food choices. Try to slow down and pay attention to what you're eating. Visualize it providing your body with the nutrients it needs to perform. Think about what the foods you eat are contributing to your overall health. Make each meal a positive experience and fortify your desire to eat healthy!

WEEK 6 🦋 DAY 6

Today's Thin Thought: A carbohydrate a day keeps the blues away.

Your daily assignments:
- **Drink lots of water.**
- **Bend, stretch, and move upon waking.**

- Walk in the morning for at least twenty-five minutes.
- Keep track of what you put in your mouth.
- Watch your servings/portions.
- Watch your intake of unhealthy fats.
- Move more during the day.
- Choose a variety of whole foods over fragmented foods.
- Take a good multivitamin/multimineral.
- Enhance your diet with nutritional supplements.

SETTING THE DAY FOR SUCCESS

Today we'll be talking about the last of our four key brain chemicals—serotonin. This neurotransmitter produces feelings of well-being, calm, and satisfaction. It's a wonderful substance! We use it constantly throughout the day to maintain emotional stability and, where our appetites are concerned, to feel full.

Serotonin is derived from tryptophan, an amino acid. When tryptophan enters the brain, it triggers the production of serotonin. If we don't have enough tryptophan, or if we are using our serotonin reserve at too high a rate, we feel anxious, irritable, and hungry. Too often, the food we crave at this point is something sugary—a carbohydrate. There is a very good reason why carbohydrates are favorite comfort foods.

In *The Serotonin Solution* by Judith J. Wurtman Ph.D. and Susan Suffes, Dr. Wurtman does a wonderful job outlining why these cravings exist. Her research over fifteen years at the Massachusetts Institute of Technology (MIT) indicates a connection between the consumption of carbohydrates and the production of serotonin. How, you may ask, can eating carbohydrates help produce something that comes from a protein? The answer speaks to the intricate way our brains work.

When we consume food with a high amount of carbohydrates and a small amount of protein, more tryptophan enters the brain than if we eat something with moderate amounts of protein and carbohydrates. This was puzzling to the researchers, whose initial thought was the more protein consumed—with the amino acids including tryptophan—the more serotonin should be produced. The opposite was true. More tryptophan was absorbed in the brain when less protein was eaten. The missing piece to this puzzle was found in the function of insulin, in response to the high degree of carbohydrates.

Tryptophan has to compete in the bloodstream for what Dr. Wurtman calls "space" to get into the brain. Because tryptophan is the least abundant of all the amino acids, when you eat protein, it has to compete with its numerous siblings. There's less room and tryptophan gets nudged out, making tryptophan like the runt of the litter. But something very special happens when you eat foods high in carbohydrates, like sugar and starch. The rush of carbohydrates stimulates the production of insulin, which enters the bloodstream in response. This insulin "pushes" amino acids, of which there is always a supply in the bloodstream, into muscle cells. There is only one amino acid insulin doesn't "push" into the muscle cells—tryptophan. With all of the other amino acids cleared out of the way into the muscle cells, the pathway is free and clear for the tryptophan to have unfettered access to the brain. When it enters the brain, serotonin is produced.[2] Thus having that sugary or

2. Wurtman, Susan, Ph.D. and Susan Suffes. *The Serotonin Solution: The Potent Substance That Can Help You Stop Bingeing, Lose Weight, and Feel Great.* New York: Fawcett Columbine, 1996.

starchy snack, when you feel tense or down, produces an initial cascade of serotonin and you feel better, at least for a while.

The only carbohydrate Dr. Wurtman found that did not produce a serotonin response was fruit. The sugar found in fruit—fructose—must first be converted by the liver into glucose before it can be used by the body. Because of this, very little insulin is released, without the resulting serotonin burst due to increased tryptophan absorption.[3] Serotonin is certainly important in its own right, but it also acts as a controller for the other neurotransmitters and hormones we've talked about this week that influence so many areas of our lives: when and how we feel physically full and satisfied with what we eat; how we sleep; our response to pain, both physical and emotional; what mood we're in and for how long; how much energy we have and our general sense of motivation. Often, how we feel physically and emotionally comes down to the interplay of serotonin, acting as a hub for biochemical activity. When serotonin is in proper balance, so are we.

There are other ways to boost your body's ability to produce serotonin. At The Center, we use a product called 5-HTP (5-hydroxytryptamine), which can be used by the body to make tryptophan. This additional supply can be utilized by the body to help maintain a more consistent supply of serotonin, resulting in improved mood and sleep.

SUCCESS IN ACTION
In your journal, I want you to think about the cravings you have. When do they occur? Is there a pattern? Do you crave certain types of food? What are

3. Ibid, page 21.

your favorite crave foods? How long do you feel better after eating? Write down your top-five favorite crave foods. Note how often you eat them, whether daily, weekly, or seasonally. In women, PMS can produce these cravings, as can SAD (seasonal affective disorder). Your cravings may be related to a specific day of the week, perhaps when your work or family stress is especially high. Be aware of how you react and what cravings you might have during holidays or near a deadline.

WEEK 6 🦋 DAY 7

Today's Thin Thought: Good food is brain food.

- Drink lots of water.
- Bend, stretch, and move upon waking.
- Walk in the morning for at least twenty-five minutes.
- Keep track of what you put in your mouth.
- Watch your servings/portions.
- Watch your intake of unhealthy fats.
- Move more during the day.
- Choose a variety of whole foods over fragmented foods.
- Take a good multivitamin/multimineral.
- Enhance your diet with nutritional supplements.

Weekly Assignment:
- Go grocery shopping for next week.

SETTING THE DAY FOR SUCCESS

We've come to the end of your crash course in brain chemistry! The important point to remember is that how you feel is not merely an emotional response but a physical reaction to life, to stress, and to what you eat. People I have worked with have been discouraged about their seeming inability to alter their anxiety or cravings. Convinced their failure is a lack of willpower, they beat themselves up for their inability to meet the challenge successfully. Many of them are successful in other areas of their life and cannot understand why they can't force their bodies to respond the way they want them to. Over time, they become more and more frustrated, sure the problem lies in their mind.

Yes, as we've seen, there can be emotional issues holding us back; but many of our obstacles come from physical syndromes. That's why in the *Thin Over 40* program we stress the benefits of physical exercise, proper hydration, healthy eating, and augmenting nutritional deficiencies with supplements. It's amazing what happens when you give the body what it needs to function, because our bodies are amazing, even over forty!

SUCCESS IN ACTION

As you go grocery shopping this week, I want you to evaluate each item you put in your cart and how it will affect your brain. After all, your brain is the conductor of a symphony of hormonal and chemical interactions. When you feed it properly, it responds with a virtuoso performance of grace and harmony. Better still, make out a shopping list right now and note what positive affects each item will have. And it's fine to include a small amount of ice cream or a package of cookies, realizing that these are to be savored sparingly during the week. Remember to choose foods that are rich in flavor and texture. Too often, we devour food without really experiencing its taste. Unsatisfied, we continue to eat and eat until we're stuffed. Rather, choose foods today that you can enjoy, relax with, and relish. Eat less but eat better.

HERO OF THE WEEK

I'd like to introduce you to a very special woman. Her name is Sandra and I first met her in 1999. Sandra came to see me because she thought she was suffering from depression. Her appetite was off; she never seemed fully rested; her moods fluctuated back and forth, from good to bad to indifferent. Some days she knew something was wrong but just didn't seem to care, opting instead to stay in bed, complaining of vague physical ailments. She'd tried antidepressants, but one made her nauseated and the other made her feel completely lethargic. Nearing a half century of life, Sarah wasn't looking forward to the next fifty feeling the way she was.

When I suggested she begin to take tryptophan to increase her production of serotonin, Sandra was skeptical. She'd never even heard of serotonin, much less tryptophan! Her knowledge of how to deal with her symptoms were pharmaceutical, not biochemical. If she ate too much, she took an appetite suppressant. When she wasn't resting properly, she took a sleeping pill. Cranky or irritable, she took Valium or Midol if it was that time of the month. All of her solutions were to mask the symptoms, not deal with them. Frankly, Sandra knew a lot about what she was feeling but very little about why.

A little fearful at first, Sandra agreed to try the tryptophan, as well as change her eating habits to include more complex carbohydrates in conjunction with protein. Over the course of several weeks, her mind began to clear from its persistent fuzziness. Her moods stabilized and she commented that her emotional reactions to events were returning to normal.

It wasn't such an effort to get out of bed in the morning. Eating healthier and exercising didn't seem like such a chore.

Sandra is my Hero of the Week because she had the courage to recognize that something wasn't right, fight (even herself) to get help, and then be open to a solution that hadn't crossed her mind. In the process, she got her mind back—not a temporary symptom-driven solution but a return of her own brain operating properly. She's learning more about herself and feeling a sense of control over her body and mind she hasn't felt in a very long time. Now, the prospect of the next fifty years seems a whole lot brighter!

Week 7
Making the Most of Rest

Week 7 🦋 Day 1

Today's Thin Thought: Early to bed, early to rise, makes a man healthy, wealthy, and wise.

Today, acknowledge to yourself that you've made it to the halfway point in your *Thin over 40* training! This is very exciting because it shows the depth of your commitment. Living healthy truly is a lifelong endeavor, whose benefits will continue to produce longevity, peace, and improved health for years to come. No quick-fix diet can do that for you. I applaud your willingness to work through these issues and implement needed changes in your life!

Those of us over forty are very familiar with today's Thin Thought, credited to one of America's founding fathers, Benjamin Franklin. We're old enough to recognize the wisdom behind that statement. But as we reach forty and beyond, it doesn't always seem to be true when it comes to the quality of our sleep. We may go to bed early, exhausted, and wake up early, still feeling tired and rundown. The truth is, there's nothing wrong with Ben's statement; what's wrong is our sleep! What Ben told us over two hundred years ago was that a productive day comes from getting a good night's sleep. What we never were told was how hard that was going to be over forty! Many of us have found the amount and quality of our sleep has degraded as we've gotten older. This week, we're going to talk about how to create, achieve, and maintain restful, restorative sleep.

Your daily assignments:
- **Drink lots of water.** Make it early enough in your day so you don't compromise your sleep!
- **Bend, stretch, and move upon waking.** Getting better sleep will help you have more energy to do this.
- **Walk in the morning for at least thirty minutes.** Half an hour is a good, round figure—that will help you avoid the same.
- **Keep track of what you put in your mouth.** By now you should be making healthier, wiser choices.
- **Watch your servings/portions.** And be sure to eat the bulk of your calories earlier in the day, when your metabolism is higher.
- **Watch your intake of unhealthy fats.** Look for better alternatives, like olive and canola oils.
- **Move more during the day.** Make it as much of a routine as your doughnut, sugary snack, or coffee used to be.
- **Choose a variety of whole foods over fragmented foods.** Continue your search for taste, texture, and flavor through natural foods.
- **Take a good multivitamin/multimineral.**
- **Enhance your diet with nutritional supplements.**
- **Intentionally pursue a good night's sleep.**

SETTING THE DAY FOR SUCCESS
This week, Setting the Day for Success is going to be about setting the *night* for success. After all, you

know how hard it is to have an active, productive day when you've had a lousy time sleeping the night before. You can't concentrate, you're lethargic, and all you can think about is sneaking off somewhere to take a nap. Everything about your day just seems to take more effort than usual. It generally puts you into survival mode, where you'll do the bare minimum, just to get out the door and back in bed. You're grumpy, you're grouchy, and even your body seems to hurt more as everyday aches and pains are magnified. Given half a chance, you'd love to call in sick and spend the day trying to catch up on the night. This isn't any way to live!

Even though there is a biological trigger for sleep—melatonin—produced by the pituitary gland during hours of darkness, we can do a lot to mess up that process. One of the prime ways is to overstimulate ourselves in the evening hours, overriding our body's natural inclination toward slowing down and preparing for sleep. For some people, even the idea of *rest* is foreign. There is awake and there is sleep, with no transition in between. While this might seem to be a productive way of thinking, it can actually rob you of the ability to perform.

C. Leslie Charles looks at some of the reasons our lives become complicated and stressful in her book, *Why Is Everyone So Cranky?*.[1] Two are particularly relevant to those of us over forty—too much to do in too little time, and the way technology has taken over lives. Let's start by looking at the first one—this idea that we have too much to do and too little time. With a mind-set like this, is it any wonder we try to cram and stuff each minute of our waking hours with ac-

1. Charles, Leslie C. *Why Is Everyone So Cranky: The Ten Trends Complicating Our Lives and What We Can Do About Them.* New York: Hyperion, 2001.

tivity? Overwhelmed by our to-do list, we end up operating on a schedule segmented into minute increments. Relaxation is considered an unattainable luxury. We simply have too much to do to waste timing relaxing. So we power our way through the day, accelerating at breakneck speed to get everything done, and then expect to slam on the brakes when our heads touch the pillow and fall asleep. This isn't reasonable.

Thanks to technology responding to our desire to make "every second count," we are caught in a trap of our own devices. With cell phones, text messaging, the Internet, e-mail, and voice mail, not only are we accessible to others 24/7, but information and tasks are accessible to us. We are losing the concept of "down time." We used to put certain tasks off because we simply couldn't do them, given the time. Now we're nudged to do one more thing no matter the time of day or night—because we can. We can even answer work voice mail or pay our bills online at three in the morning. What started out as a convenience, for some, has turned into a compulsion. It was meant to make our lives easier and instead has created a nightmare of unending expectations.

SUCCESS IN ACTION

In your journal today, I'd like you to evaluate how your time is spent during the day. Think specifically about the amount of time, and when, you give yourself permission to relax. Do you take a few minutes in the morning to read over the paper or watch a television show prior to going to work? Do you consider your stretching and walking each morning to be a form of relaxation? Do you approach them that way? Or as just another task you're completing? During the day do you stop and take a break during lunch, to relax?

Or do you grab bites in between tasks, while sitting at your desk surrounded by a cacophony of activity? In the late evening, how do you relax? Do you quietly read a book or watch television?

All of us need to take time during each day to slow down the pace and give our minds and our bodies a break from the constant barrage of responsibilities and duties we are called on to perform. Evaluate today whether or not you're factoring in time for yourself.

WEEK 7   🦋   DAY 2

Today's Thin Thought: Sleep is not a waste of time.

Your daily assignments:
- **Drink lots of water.**
- **Bend, stretch, and move upon waking.**
- **Walk in the morning for at least thirty minutes.**
- **Keep track of what you put in your mouth.**
- **Watch your servings/portions.**
- **Watch your intake of unhealthy fats.**
- **Move more during the day.**
- **Choose a variety of whole foods over fragmented foods.**
- **Take a good multivitamin/multimineral.**
- **Enhance your diet with nutritional supplements.**
- **Intentionally pursue a good night's sleep.**

SETTING THE DAY FOR SUCCESS

You may be asking yourself, "Why an entire week on sleep?" Frankly, many people are biased against sleep. They see it as an unwelcome invasion into their productive awake time. Therefore, they make excuses for not getting enough sleep. Sleep does not seem that important.

I've always been interested in sleep patterns and sleep deprivation. In college, one of my jobs was at a university research laboratory in Seattle, observing those having trouble achieving restful, restorative sleep. I learned that even though a person "sleeps" for the recommended seven to eight hours a night, the quality of that sleep might be so compromised that they wake up fatigued, irritable, and functioning at a subnormal level. Rarely did people in their twenties come in. Mostly, it was those approaching or past the age of forty.

When you're younger, it just doesn't seem to be that much of a problem to cheat yourself of sleep. Shaving off hours of sleep each night seemed to be the normal course of things. Over forty, this habit becomes harder and harder to pull off, just at the time when our lives have never seemed more compacted with things to do. We tell ourselves that it's worth not getting a good night's sleep in order to get this or that done. But is it worth it, especially as a regular habit?

Contrary to the idea that sleep is a time of inactivity, there's a lot going on while our bodies are sleeping. It's the time when we're actively involved in repair and maintenance of large and small injuries and insults. During sleep, the body produces high levels of human growth hormone (HGH), which corrects damage to our cells and helps promote the formation of lean muscle tissue. During sleep, our brains are also sorting and organizing all of the information it's had to process during the day. You could consider it kind of a nightly "defrag" of your brain.

It's time we gave sleep, and by extension ourselves, more respect.

SUCCESS IN ACTION

Today I'd like you to write about your history with sleep. Think back over the course of your life and examine how your attitudes or even your sleeping habits themselves have changed as you've aged. Do you remember enjoying sleep as a child? Do you wish you could sleep that way again? Is sleep a time where you feel "unsafe?" If so, can you identify why you feel that way? Write three short paragraphs: (1) How I slept as a child; (2) How I slept as a young adult; and (3) How I sleep now. If you've experienced sleep degradation, begin to identify reasons. If you've always been a good sleeper, and still are, take this week to appreciate this positive aspect in your life! Recommit to maintaining the habits that help you sustain restful sleep.

WEEK 7   🦋   DAY 3

Today's Thin Thought: A good night's sleep can help you lose weight.

Your daily assignments:
   • **Drink lots of water.**
   • **Bend, stretch, and move upon waking.**
   • **Walk in the morning for at least thirty minutes.**
   • **Keep track of what you put in your mouth.**
   • **Watch your servings/portions.**
   • **Watch your intake of unhealthy fats.**
   • **Move more during the day.**
   • **Choose a variety of whole foods over fragmented foods.**
   • **Take a good multivitamin/multimineral.**

- Enhance your diet with nutritional supplements.
- Intentionally pursue a good night's sleep.

Your weekly assignment:
- Weigh yourself.

SETTING THE DAY FOR SUCCESS

Today is the day you weigh yourself. How well you sleep has a direct effect on your weight maintenance and weight loss. If you are tired, you don't feel like exercising or even moving much, for that matter. If you're sleeping poorly, you may spend a greater number of hours either sleeping or napping, during which your body needs fewer calories. Your metabolism goes down and you burn fewer calories.

It's important to get your rest. Many people use food to jump-start a lethargic, tired body. Instead of getting enough rest to feel good during the day, they use high-calorie foods and caffeinated beverages to boost their energy. Not only is this method short-lived, it adds calories and pounds. It's time to give sleep the respect it's due and give yourself the time you need to wind down in the evening and go to sleep.

This does not mean I'm advocating a return to the couch potato after dinner. On the contrary, exercise in the early evening positions your body to relax later on. It actually contributes to your ability to sleep, so don't worry about that walk or playtime with the kids! But after you've had your physical activity in the evening, you need to begin to prepare yourself for sleep.

Remember, sleep is brought about by the production of melatonin during the hours of darkness. How many of us, though, keep the lights blaring, the television or radio blasting, or sit nose to nose with the computer screen, right up until the time we go to bed? Is it any wonder we have trouble getting to sleep or toss and turn all night? And after a night like that, who wants to get up early to make sure you can stretch and exercise in the morning before work? It's an effort even to get up in order to get to work on time.

SUCCESS IN ACTION

For the rest of this week, I want you to be intentional about how you are going to prepare for sleep. I want you to write down the proactive steps you take to get ready. Factor in when you need to get up in the morning so you can be sure you have seven to eight hours of sleep set aside. You'll want to start earlier than that in the evening by reducing the light level, noise level, and activity level. Your action plan for rest will need to factor in any other members of your household. You can set the tone for the evening by slowing yourself down and giving your body time to transition into a good night's sleep.

Write down five specific things you are going to do the rest of this week to facilitate the rest your body needs. It can be anything from giving yourself permission to sit and read a book for half an hour before going to bed, to putting on relaxing music or nature sounds to encourage your mind to relax. It could be taking a hot bath or spending some time in a Jacuzzi or hot tub, if you have one available. It could be enjoying a burst of activity in the early evening to encourage your body to relax later on. Think about your particular situation and prepare for this vital, restorative activity.

WEEK 7 🦋 DAY 4

Today's Thin Thought: If your mind's racing,
your body can't slow down.

Your daily assignments:
- Drink lots of water.
- Bend, stretch, and move upon waking.
- Walk in the morning for at least thirty minutes.
- Keep track of what you put in your mouth.
- Watch your servings/portions.
- Watch your intake of unhealthy fats.
- Move more during the day.
- Choose a variety of whole foods over fragmented foods.
- Take a good multivitamin/multimineral.
- Enhance your diet with nutritional supplements.
- Intentionally pursue a good night's sleep.

SETTING THE DAY FOR SUCCESS

It's difficult for your body to rest and sleep if your mind is stuck on fast-forward. I'm sure most of you have experienced the sleep disturbances that come prior to the start of a family trip, an important business meeting, or even an anticipated confrontation with a friend or associate. Your body may be dog tired, but your mind won't quit going over and over the details of the upcoming event. Even in the case of something eagerly anticipated, such as a vacation, you can't sleep. You worry about the alarm not going off and sleeping through your flight. You worry whether you've left all the necessary instructions for the neighbor who's watching the house. You worry that you've forgotten to pack some vital item. The bottom line is you worry.

Worry robs us of sleep. It is an often strenuous mental activity that rarely produces any beneficial insight or unforeseen solution. Yet still we do it. In order to get the rest we require, we need to stop. That, of course, can be easier said than done. Worry rises out of a concern of being unprepared or a fear of a negative consequence. You may have missed your flight two years ago or left your speech notes on the kitchen table or remember how badly your last confrontation went with that person. All those things would seem to whisper that your concern and worry is justified. The problem is, all that whispering keeps you up at night!

It is possible to take steps that guard against the negative consequences. For example, if you're worried about not hearing the alarm, you can get a louder, more obnoxious alarm clock, or you can position several alarms throughout the room on the theory that even if one fails, the others will work and wake you up. If you are concerned about leaving behind something important for that business meeting, pack your car or your briefcase the night before. If you're worried how the conversation is going to go with that other person, write down the points you want to be sure to get across and give yourself permission to use those during your meeting. When you feel more in control, you will worry less.

Oftentimes, the worry you experience has nothing to do with a realistic assessment of the potential for things to go wrong. Rather, you worry because that little voice inside your head speaks from a position of negativity. You can't let go of the day because you feel you've failed in some way. You can't stop beating yourself up over a perceived failure. You can't rest because you don't feel entitled to it. The television blaring is merely your way of drowning out that voice. Darkness and quiet only seem to amplify your feelings of inadequacy. In this case, rest and sleep are not positive for you. Rather, they are times when you feel most vulnerable and under attack from your own insecurities. When the rest of the world is sleeping, you have only yourself for company.

In order to relax, that transition time between wake and sleep needs to be a positive, supportive review of your day and yourself. If you've had a great day, you need to take comfort in that, not consider it an aberration. If you've had a bad day, you need to evaluate what went wrong and why, for the purpose of learning and growing from it. It's time for you to pay attention to—and direct—the voices in your head that lull you to sleep.

SUCCESS IN ACTION

I want you to ask yourself whether you are the sort of person who has trouble "putting down" the day. Do you put it down and then immediately pick it back up again by worrying and reliving it? Do you ever feel satisfied with how the day has gone? Or do you find yourself with a constant complaint about your life that just won't go away? Have you ever used alcohol or drugs to help you sleep so you could turn off that voice in your head? Are you so consumed with what you need to do tomorrow that you can't relax and rest tonight? What do you think you're accomplishing by engaging in so much worry?

Write down the things you find yourself habitually worrying about. (If you're worrying about them all through the day, you can be sure they are invading your peace at night.) For each worry item, list three positive steps you are going to take to address the situation. If it's a situation that can't be addressed, how is worrying going to help you? When you find yourself worrying about each item, remind yourself of what you're going to do to be proactive in dealing with it. Remind yourself that you are in control of your life and your rest. Commit to reducing your habit of worrying so you can increase the quality of your sleep.

WEEK 7   🦋   DAY 5

Today's Thin Thought: You don't have to get to bed early, just get to bed on time.

Your daily assignments:
* **Drink lots of water.**
* **Bend, stretch, and move upon waking.**
* **Walk in the morning for at least thirty minutes.**
* **Keep track of what you put in your mouth.**
* **Watch your servings/portions.**
* **Watch your intake of unhealthy fats.**
* **Move more during the day.**
* **Choose a variety of whole foods over fragmented foods.**
* **Take a good multivitamin/multimineral.**
* **Enhance your diet with nutritional supplements.**
* **Intentionally pursue a good night's sleep.**

SETTING THE DAY FOR SUCCESS

As we continue our discussion this week about helping our bodies achieve restful sleep, I'd like you to think about your activity patterns during the evening. Do you go to bed early some nights yet stay up late on others? This is especially important as we head into the weekend. Some of us will get to bed at a "normal" time during the week but think of the weekend as a time when it doesn't really matter when we go to bed, as long as we sleep later to make up for it. This isn't really an issue if it happens rarely—life requires certain flexibility. But if this is your pattern on a regular basis, your sleep cycles could become disturbed.

Say you usually try to get to bed by 10:30 p.m. on weeknights but on weekends you find yourself staying up until 12:00 or 1:00 a.m. You've now extended your wake cycle by around two hours. If you sleep in to compensate, chances are you aren't going to be tired Sunday night or ready to get up Monday morning two hours earlier than you did the last two days. Two hours may not seem like much, but it is a lot when it's the difference between getting up feeling rested at 6:00 a.m. versus 8:00 a.m. or later. My recommendation is to try to stay within an hour's time frame of retiring and rising each and every day. We are creatures of habit with established biorhythms that don't know when it's Friday or Tuesday night. Try to maintain a consistent wake-sleep cycle of sixteen to seventeen hours awake followed by seven to eight hours asleep.

Each of us has had times when we've needed to stay up later than usual to accomplish some sort of task. You know the second wind you get after you've forced yourself over the line of drowsiness. Sure you can do it, but it places stress on your body to respond in this way. The younger and healthier you are, the better your body is able to handle this stress. Over forty, it becomes harder. And if you want to stay healthy, in order to be able to do this infrequently when necessary, you need to get your rest! Don't consider it a luxury—rest is a necessity!

SUCCESS IN ACTION

For the rest of this week and next, I want you to document when you go to sleep and when you wake up. When you wake may be different from when you actually get up. On your journal page for today, write down four column heads: Retire, Sleep, Wake, Get Up. In other words, I'd like you to track the time you get into bed, estimate the time you actually got to sleep, the time you first awakened (estimate if you don't know the exact time), and the time you got up.

Track how you're doing. Is there a great deal of difference from day to day? If so, why? Is it because of a job? Is it because of an activity? Is it simply a choice you're making? If you have not established a fairly consistent routine, what would it take to do so? Do you perceive the benefits of changing your pattern to outweigh any negatives? If you are consistently cheating yourself of sleep, why? How are those activities more important than your health?

WEEK 7 ❧ DAY 6

Today's Thin Thought: When it comes to sleep, think quantity and quality.

Your daily assignments:

- **Drink lots of water.**
- **Bend, stretch, and move upon waking.**
- **Walk in the morning for at least thirty minutes.**
- **Keep track of what you put in your mouth.**
- **Watch your servings/portions.**
- **Watch your intake of unhealthy fats.**
- **Move more during the day.**
- **Choose a variety of whole foods over fragmented foods.**
- **Take a good multivitamin/multimineral.**

- **Enhance your diet with nutritional supplements.**
- **Intentionally pursue a good night's sleep.**

SETTING THE DAY FOR SUCCESS

As we age, our muscles and tissues can lose tautness. Simply put, they can get flabby. And it's not just the muscles we see but can also be internal. This flabbiness of internal tissue can cause one of the greatest thieves of sleep, stamina, and good health. It's called sleep apnea. As a sleep technician, I have seen the deleterious effects of this condition. At its most severe form, it can be life threatening. No, sleep isn't something any of us should take for granted.

Sleep comes in five stages, from light (Stage 1) to REM (Stage 5, which is when we dream). According to data from the National Sleep Foundation, about half of our sleep time is in Stage 2, or medium, sleep. Stages 3 and 4 are categorized as deep sleep, and take up about 20 to 25 percent of our sleep time. We spend another 20 to 25 percent in Stage 5 sleep, and the rest in Stage 1 sleep, moving in and out between wake and sleep.[2] Age can compromise the ability to reach and maintain Stage 5, or REM, sleep.

Everyone's throat will relax during sleep. When it relaxes to the point that the upper tissue closes down on the lower tissue, snoring occurs. (The sound is produced by the air being pulled by the lungs through a restricted space.) With sleep apnea, those tissues close off completely, allowing no air to pass through. You stop breathing. In response, the body initiates a gasping reflex that opens up the air passages but also wakes you up. Although you'll rarely

2. Seven, Richard. "Eyes Wide Shut: The night life that shapes us," *Seattle Times, Pacific Northwest Magazine*, June 6, 2003, page 31.

remember being awakened, you have been jerked out of deeper sleep into wakefulness and must go back through the process all over again. This back and forth, in and out of sleep, is very stressful on the body and leads to weight gain and daytime tiredness, as well as reduced oxygenation during sleep. This constant state of fatigue puts a tremendous strain on all of the major organs of the body, including the heart. This isn't inconvenient, it's very serious.

SUCCESS IN ACTION

I'd like you to reflect today on what a gift good sleep is to your body. It's time to put rest and sleep in the same category our bodies do—as critical to our health, stamina, and quality of life. If you are having difficulty getting a good night's sleep and you believe that there may be a physical cause, such as excessive snoring or sleep apnea, your assignment today is to contact your primary-care physician, hospital, or sleep clinic and make an appointment to consult with a medical professional. Do it today. Apnea is a serious medical condition that needs to be addressed.

WEEK 7 🦋 DAY 7

Today's Thin Thought: The best therapy is common sense.

Your daily assignments:
- **Drink lots of water.**
- **Bend, stretch, and move upon waking.**
- **Walk in the morning for at least thirty minutes.**
- **Keep track of what you put in your mouth.**
- **Watch your servings/portions.**
- **Watch your intake of unhealthy fats.**

- Move more during the day.
- Choose a variety of whole foods over fragmented foods.
- Take a good multivitamin/multimineral.
- Enhance your diet with nutritional supplements.
- Intentionally pursue a good night's sleep.

Weekly Assignment:
- Go grocery shopping for next week.

SETTING THE DAY FOR SUCCESS

The Thin Thought for today comes from Dr. Michael Vitiello, a psychiatry and behavioral sciences professor at the University of Washington, and a senior scientist with the Sleep Research Group.[3] In a recent article in the *Seattle Times*, he listed some steps you can take to improve your sleep. I want you to see them because they will support what you've learned already this week and provide you with another voice on how important this aspect of your life is. Paraphrased, here are Dr. Vitiello's tips:

- As much as you can, keep to a regular sleep schedule.
- Get enough sleep each night. If you don't, you'll have trouble repaying your sleep debt.
- Prepare your environment. Keep it dark, quiet, a comfortable temperature, with a comfortable mattress and good air flow.
- Don't drink or smoke from the late afternoon on. Cigarettes are a stimulant and alcohol adversely affects sleep quality.
- Keep your bedroom a sanctuary. Don't keep a television, a computer, or a desk in there.

3. Ibid, page 34.

- Having trouble sleeping? Try warm milk. It has properties that help you sleep.
- If you can't get to sleep, turn the clock around. It won't help just watching and thinking about how late it's getting.
- Exercise during the day and expose yourself to light.
- If it helps, take a warm bath or shower in the evening.[4]

If you'll permit me to add to Dr. Vitiello's list, there is another step you can take to improve the quality of your sleep. It is 5-HTP. This is the supplement I mentioned last week that assists in the supply of serotonin to the brain. Serotonin is what is called a precursor to melatonin, the substance produced by your pituitary during hours of darkness that triggers your brain to sleep. If your body is compromised in its ability to produce enough melatonin to encourage a healthy sleep cycle, we have found 5-HTP to be of great help. I encourage you to go online and read about this supplement on www.thinover40.com, or speak to a health care professional. We have found this supplement to be a much better alternative than alcohol or sleeping pills.

SUCCESS IN ACTION

It is my hope that you've come to appreciate the proper place rest and sleep should have in your *Thin over 40* life. In order to be as active and healthy as you desire, you've got to invest in your body through restorative sleep. I'd like you to document any changes you need to make to your sleeping environment. If you do not sleep alone, it will be a positive reinforcement for you to explain to your sleeping

4. Ibid.

partner why these changes are so necessary. Enact as many of them as you can, even if it means moving a television or going to the store to buy light-reducing blinds. If your bed is not comfortable, take steps to make it more so or consider purchasing a new mattress altogether. Spend as much as you are able on the best-quality mattress you can buy. There really is a difference, and you want a mattress that is going to help you get a good night's sleep.

Read back over your entries this week. If you should have set up an appointment with a physician and haven't, do so. Sleep is one of the Five Success Essentials to the *Thin over 40* lifestyle—vital to your progress! It's amazing the way the body is able to recover fairly quickly from a prolonged sleep deficit. See if you don't agree after three straight nights of restful sleep! You'll feel energized, revitalized, and more optimistic!

HERO OF THE WEEK

Robert is forty-six years old and sleeps with a CPAP machine. A CPAP machine is one that sends air under pressure through a mask and helps Robert sleep each night. Robert has sleep apnea, and if he doesn't use this machine, he can't sleep. It wasn't easy for him to admit he had a physical problem. In fact, for a year he kept waving off his wife's concerns about his snoring and breathing problems when he slept. After his wife spent months sleeping on the couch to avoid the noise of his snoring and the distraction of his gasping, Robert decided it was time to do something about it. He went in to a sleep center for a sleep study, where he was quickly diagnosed with severe apnea. In fact, on the night of the study, Robert stopped breathing an average of seventy times an hour—over once a minute! Over and over

Robert would wake himself up, gasping for air. Exhausted, he'd fall right back to sleep, to do it all over again. Robert didn't realize it, but he was at serious risk, and not only because of what was happening to him physiologically. You see, as a salesman, Robert spent a great deal of his time driving. It got to the point where he had to pull the car over in the middle of his day to nap, where the apnea would begin again. At the sleep center he learned that many people in his condition were at risk for automobile accidents, due to their extreme fatigue. Slowly, sleeping poorly night after night was stealing Robert's life.

Robert is my Hero of the Week because he accepted the reality of his condition and took steps to get help. He sleeps now, every single nap and every single night, with a mask around his face and tubing that snakes up to the CPAP machine, which whirs like a room fan. Rather than resent this facet of his life, Robert is grateful for the technology that is saving his life and doesn't complain. His wife doesn't either. She's off the couch and back in bed with Robert, and the soothing "white noise" of the machine helps *her* sleep.

If you suspect a problem like apnea, be a hero to your family and ask for the help you need. Apnea strikes both men and women. I have many female clients who are being helped by a CPAP machine or surgery to correct excessive snoring or apnea. Robert understands how important sleep is to his quality of life, and so should you!

WEEK 8
MAKING THE MOST OF "THE CHANGE"

WEEK 8 🦋 DAY 1

Today's Thin Thought: Age and guile over youth and beauty.

We're starting our eighth week of *Thin over 40*, and we're going to stop a moment and take a pause—a pause to look at the effects of aging and weight gain due to menopause in women and andropause in men. This week's Key Concept is Hormones. All of you have most likely heard of menopause, that time in a woman's life that marks the cessation of menstruation. It's euphemistically known as "the Change."

Not as well known, however, is the term andropause. As I write this, my word-processing program is screaming at me there's no such word as andropause and surely I've made a mistake. While not as widely accepted as menopause, I believe there are physiologically relevant changes that occur in a man, directly related to a drop in his production of testosterone—andropause.

In both genders, this "pause" results in an alteration in the production and ratio of the sex hormones estrogen, progesterone, and testosterone. These changes must be factored into the *Thin over 40* lifestyle.

Your daily assignments:
- **Drink lots of water.** By now this should be your primary source of fluids.
- **Bend, stretch, and move upon waking.** Very important during this week.
- **Walk in the morning for at least thirty minutes.** Keep moving forward and making progress!
- **Keep track of what you put in your mouth.** Remember, everything counts—and adds up!
- **Watch your servings/portions.** Don't eat on autopilot—slow down and enjoy your smaller portions.
- **Watch your intake of unhealthy fats.** Choose healthy fats, rich in omega-3.
- **Move more during the day.** Be consistent, be creative.
- **Choose a variety of whole foods over fragmented foods.** The less processing, the better!
- **Take a good multivitamin/multimineral.**
- **Enhance your diet with nutritional supplements.** From your multi to specialized supplements, support your body and your health.
- **Intentionally pursue a good night's sleep.** Don't skimp on this important renewing and rebuilding time.

SETTING THE DAY FOR SUCCESS

Today's Thin Thought is an oft-quoted line. People who are older use it against those who are younger. Young people hear the line and think they'd still rather be young and beautiful than old and crafty. Older people really think the same thing—oh, to be young and beautiful! In other cultures, aging is seen as gain, but in our society, aging is seen as loss. This seems especially true with menopause and andropause. They are perceived as losses—loss of vitality, loss of sexuality, loss of purpose, loss of youthful physique.

We live in a youth-obsessed culture, especially in the area of physicality. It's as if we've taken what we consider the physical prime of someone in their twenties and used it as a standard by which all other ages are judged. The young can't wait to grow up to look like that image, and those past that image obsess over ways to recapture it, if they ever had it at all. Sadly, it's often not even our own twenties we use. Instead it's some young body, heralded by the media, that we've concluded is the epitome of perfection— the model, the athlete, the celebrity. Frankly, we come off poorly by comparison. And the older we get, the more desperate we become to try to grab on to just a piece of the perfection, or else we've failed. If we haven't hit perfection by forty, we figure we never will and just quit trying. Instead of admitting defeat, maybe it's time we changed our perception of what is desirable. Instead of pursuing perfection, maybe we should mature our concept of what is valuable.

SUCCESS IN ACTION

Today I'd like you to take some time to really think about what you perceive as physical "perfection." Is it a flat stomach? A certain weight? Is it firm arms? Fitting into a certain pants size? What is perfection to you? Have you always felt that way, or have your ideals of perfection changed? What caused the change—desperation?

I know you've done this before, but I'd like you to record again just what your goals are. Now, take a look at those goals and place them up against your idea of perfection. Are they different? If they are, does one need to change?

In other words, if deep down you think only perfection equals success, and you're going to settle for less by being "realistic," how motivated can that make you to continue in the *Thin over 40* lifestyle? Perhaps you need to examine where your idea of perfection comes from and make adjustments.

If you think success is only looking like some ideal, you've created enormous room for failure. In order to succeed at most anything, you need to refocus on success. Write down realistic, attainable goals under the heading of "Success!"

WEEK 8 🦋 DAY 2

Today's Thin Thought: The Change is not a disease.

Your daily assignments:
- **Drink lots of water.**
- **Bend, stretch, and use your weights upon waking.**
- **Walk in the morning for at least thirty minutes.**
- **Keep track of what you put in your mouth.**
- **Watch your servings/portions.**
- **Watch your intake of unhealthy fats.**
- **Move more during the day.**
- **Choose a variety of whole foods over fragmented foods.**
- **Take a good multivitamin/multimineral.**
- **Enhance your diet with nutritional supplements.**
- **Intentionally pursue a good night's sleep.**

SETTING THE DAY FOR SUCCESS

The change in our hormones as we age is not a disease. It's not a condition. Yes, there are physical consequences, but those can be addressed successfully. The caveat, of course, is that addressing them takes time, patience, and perseverance. In a youth-obsessed society, we are also used to a medically proactive culture. Interpreting our aging as a negative, we demand that doctors "fix" it. If the problem is low estrogen, we want a shot to pump it up. Likewise with testosterone. Do it now, do it right, we tell our doctors. Unfortunately, it hasn't proven that easy to do.

Let's take a minute and really look at what happens during both menopause and andropause. Menopause is the ending of the menstrual cycle . . . that's it. Pretty short explanation, right? So why is it that this process seems to take forever? Just like in puberty, your body requires time to accomplish this complex hormonal dance. It took time to gear up to puberty and it takes time to gear down from menstruation. Time is an important factor in menopause, for the abruptness at which hormonal levels drop relates to the severity of menopausal symptoms, such as hot flashes, vaginal dryness, weight gain, and mood swings. Yes, you heard it right—weight gain. This is a natural part of menopause. This is why strategies that used to work in your twenties no longer do. It's not that you must resign yourself to getting bigger and bigger, but that you need to understand what is happening in your body and why.

As estrogen production begins to drop off, the female body responds by encouraging the growth of fat cells. Why? Because fat cells have the ability to produce estrogen. (For a wonderful, enlightening look at this process, I encourage you to read Debra

Waterhouse's book, *Outsmarting the Midlife Fat Cell.*[1]) Your body is attempting to compensate for the loss of estrogen through one part of your body by producing it in another—your fat cells. You may not be happy with your fat cells during menopause, but your body is. It is especially happy with abdominal fat cells, which are super estrogen producers. Your body supports what it's happy with. Thus, when you put on weight during menopause, it is concentrated around the abdominal area. Your waistline expands.

During this time of menopause, you will also have a drop in progesterone production. Progesterone is highest in the body after ovulation. As menopause approaches, you will have times when your period happens without ovulation occurring first (anovulation). During anovulation, estrogen and progesterone levels can be extremely erratic, with dramatic dips and rises. Progesterone, which is released upon ovulation, counterbalances estrogen. But if ovulation does not occur, your progesterone level declines, leading to an overabundance of estrogen in the body. When estrogen spikes, you may experience mood swings, water retention, weight gain (again!), problems sleeping, breast swelling and/or tenderness.

You men, who are now thanking your lucky stars you were not born female and thus avoided these problems, might want to hold on just a bit. Men also experience a drop in hormone production and an alteration in their balance of the sex hormones testosterone, progesterone, and estrogen. This loss, or andropause, can lead to symptoms such as a loss of lean muscle with a corresponding rise in fat, especially around the middle. Night urination is a symp-

1. Waterhouse, Debra, MPH, RD. *Outsmarting the Midlife Fat Cell: Winning Weight Control Strategies for Women over 35 to Stay Fit Through Menopause.* New York: Hyperion, 1999.

tom, as are thinning and graying hair, and an increase in prostate size. Perhaps the symptom most disturbing to men is the reduction in their libido, or interest and ability to perform sexually.

Maybe it's not time to gloat just yet. Perhaps it is time to have empathy, compassion, and care for each other as we collectively maneuver through this time in our lives.

SUCCESS IN ACTION

Face it—"the Change," whether male or female, is a fact of life. Pretending it doesn't exist, or considering it a dreaded state of being, isn't helpful. What is helpful is to understand the physical mechanics, gain new respect for your body, and discover ways to assist your body through this natural process.

Make a timeline today, of the significant events in your life. Be honest about them. Indicate the negatives you learned from and the positives you gained from. Go back to your birth and chart the memorable things that have happened to you and that you've participated in. Under each, leave space for "What I've Gained" or "Lessons Learned." (You are not allowed under "What I've Gained" to just put weight!) Go all the way up to today. Think also about what you've gained and learned over the past seven-plus weeks. Write them out and celebrate your success. This time in your life is significant, but it doesn't have to be drenched in negatives. Your body may have a certain agenda, but you can work with it to be the very best possible.

Take a minute to project what milestones you have to look forward to in the future. This is a wonderful time to recommit to becoming healthy and happy, to make the most of those times to come. Your *Thin over*

40 life does not lament the years past—it looks forward to your full life ahead!

WEEK 8   🦋   DAY 3

*Today's Thin Thought: Make peace with your
body as you age.*

Your daily assignments:
- **Drink lots of water.**
- **Bend, stretch, and use your weights upon
waking.**
- **Walk in the morning for at least thirty
minutes.**
- **Keep track of what you put in your mouth.**
- **Watch your servings/portions.**
- **Watch your intake of unhealthy fats.**
- **Move more during the day.**
- **Choose a variety of whole foods over frag-
mented foods.**
- **Take a good multivitamin/multimineral.**
- **Enhance your diet with nutritional supple-
ments.**
- **Intentionally pursue a good night's sleep.**

Your weekly assignment:
- **Weigh yourself.**

SETTING THE DAY FOR SUCCESS

Over the next several days, we're going to concentrate on positive, proactive steps men and women
can take to improve this hormonal transition into
middle age. Whether you are a man or a woman,
take a look at these suggestions. You may be surprised that many of them can apply to both.

Both men and women can benefit from an increase

in physical activity. Because both menopause and andropause result in a loss of lean muscle, metabolism can decrease. Cardiovascular exercise, such as walking, jogging, biking, or swimming, helps promote higher metabolic levels. There is also another kind of exercise that is very beneficial. It is often called "strength training." This exercise is not primarily cardiovascular in nature, but rather, builds lean muscle mass. Strength training specifically targets the addition of muscle tissue through resistance work. It places stress on your muscles, which respond by strengthening themselves and increasing in size.

If you don't exercise, the muscle you do have will be replaced with fat. For women and men, more muscle means a higher metabolism, a firmer, toned body, and greater strength for daily activities. For men, physical exercise is an important component in testosterone production, and not just for younger men. Testosterone levels in middle-aged men also elevate after exercise.[2]

Strength training doesn't necessarily need to happen in a gym. Working around the house or yard can turn into strength training if you're using your muscles. You want to make sure to work all muscle groups, like your back, arms, and chest. Walking is especially good for the buttocks and legs.

You've got a great start stretching and using your weights in the morning. For those of you looking to do more, consider becoming part of a local recreation center or gym, where there is a variety of weights to choose from. You will also have access to personnel

2. Kraemer W.J., et al. "Effects of Heavy-Resistance Training on Hormonal Response Patterns in Younger Vs. Older Men." *J App Physiol* (1999) 87, 3: 982–92, as referenced in "Male Menopause" by Edward D. Rosick, *Life Extension* magazine, October 2003, page 69.

who are familiar with the weights and with the proper way to use them. If you can find a friend to go with you, all the better!

In order to safeguard the muscle you have and gain more, you need to engage in activities that use them—hence the warning "use it or lose it." In order to keep your metabolism up, you need to engage in strength training and cardiovascular activity. If all of this seems like a bother and a waste of time, remember it is our time-saving propensity that has factored out these types of normal daily activities. These used to be a part of life, until we became efficient at eliminating them. Whether we like it or not, we're going to have to intentionally integrate more physicality into our routines! Our bodies were meant to move and stretch, bend and reach, walk and breathe deeply.

SUCCESS IN ACTION

In your journal today, I want you to write down your plan for incorporating strength training three times per week. Ideally you want to have a day off between each training day in order to give your muscles time to repair. When you strength train, you put stress on the muscles. They respond by repairing themselves stronger than they were before by adding muscle tissue. In this way, you gain new muscle. Remember, if you do nothing, you will lose muscle mass through "the Change." And when you reduce muscle mass, you put out the fat-burning fire that lean muscle represents. Your metabolism slows down and fat builds up.

If you find yourself hesitating about adding this to your *Thin over 40* lifestyle, I want you to be honest about why. What do you think will happen if you do? What are you fearful or apprehensive about? Is it the time involved? Do you doubt this will be beneficial? Do you have a vision of yourself barely able to lift a set of free weights? Is it pride? What is causing a stumbling block for you? Where does it come from? Write down your specific objections. Now, look at them and come up with an answer, a way around them. If the roadblock is time, look over your schedule and find twenty minutes three times a week. (If your schedule is so full you can't find those twenty-minute slots, it's too full! Think of it another way; you find time to eat, to run errands, to watch that television show, or hop on the computer. What you *really* value, you find time to do. It's time you valued your health and your life.) If the roadblock is skepticism, commit to conducting an experiment to determine how effective strength training can actually be. If it's fear of going to a gym and looking foolish, invest in a set of free weights for your spare room, basement, or garage and lift in private. Whatever the objection, find a way around it! Remember, one of your sessions could be on the weekends, doing yard work or some other project that involves using your muscles. Building strength and toning your muscles will allow you to feel better, look better, and help you navigate the passage through menopause or andropause.

WEEK 8 ❦ DAY 4

Today's Thin Thought: Estrogen isn't only a woman's hormone.

Your daily assignments:
- **Drink lots of water.**
- **Bend, stretch, and use your weights upon waking.**
- **Walk in the morning for at least thirty minutes.**

- Keep track of what you put in your mouth.
- Watch your servings/portions.
- Watch your intake of unhealthy fats.
- Move more during the day.
- Choose a variety of whole foods over fragmented foods.
- Take a good multivitamin/multimineral.
- Enhance your diet with nutritional supplements.
- Intentionally pursue a good night's sleep.

SETTING THE DAY FOR SUCCESS

Say the word "estrogen" and most people automatically think of women. True, estrogen is one of the main female hormones. During menopause, estrogen levels can drop, causing menopausal symptoms. If progesterone production drops even more, the estrogen-progesterone balance can skew, causing an overabundance of estrogen in the system. Out-of-balance estrogen can have negative effects in women. It can also have negative effects in men.

In *The Testosterone Syndrome* by Eugene Shippen, M.D., and William Fryer,[3] Dr. Shippen gives seven reasons for elevated estrogen levels in men during middle age. The first is the very act of aging, which increases male production of a substance—aromatase—that converts testosterone to estrogen. The second is an increased middle-age load on the liver. Part of the liver's job is to remove excess estrogen from the body. If liver function is compromised, it doesn't do its job as effectively and more estrogen

3. Shippen, Eugene, M.D., and William Fryer. *The Testosterone Syndrome. The Critical Factor for Energy, Health, & Sexuality—Reversing the Male Menopause.* New York: M. Evans and Company, 1998.

stays in the body. Third, add to that zinc deficiency. Zinc is used by the body in sperm and testosterone production. If zinc is low, sexual functioning is compromised.

Fourth: Remember the abdominal fat cells? Excess weight produces estrogen, whether you are male or female. In men, obesity causes a loss of testosterone and an increase in estrogen. Fifth, there is alcohol use. Alcohol, which must be processed as a toxin by the liver, puts added strain on that organ and decreases levels of zinc. The sixth effect, drug-induced estrogen imbalance, is also linked to zinc deficiencies. Dr. Shippen notes that the common use of diuretics to reduce male hypertension has the undesirable side effect of leeching zinc from the body. The seventh and last cause he notes is an insidious one—eating estrogen-producing foods or being exposed to estrogenlike substances in our environment.[4]

For both men and women, I cannot stress enough the need to reduce excess body fat. Again, that is *excess* body fat. Women, especially, need a certain amount of fat to assist in estrogen production as menstruation ceases. However, it becomes very important as both men and women age to keep fat from forming. Usually, this fat is kept near the abdomen, in abdominal fat cells. The increase in weight at the waist produces the apple shape so common in older men and women. Unfortunately, this type of body shape has been shown to increase the risk for heart-related disorders over the pear body shape, where the majority of fat is deposited on the hips and legs.

An expanding waistline is cause for action. But it's more than just vanity that should propel you to maintain your commitment to living *Thin over 40*.

4. Ibid, pages 50–52.

This isn't about physical perfection or an Adonis physique. This is a life and health issue!

SUCCESS IN ACTION
—If you're a man, think about the factors listed that put you at risk for a testosterone/estrogen imbalance. The first you can't do anything about—you cannot stop aging. But look at the rest of the list. Perhaps you can make proactive changes to slow the effects of aging.

• Be kind to your liver. Decrease the amount of toxins you expose yourself to in order to cut down on the amount it has to filter out each day.
• Take a supplement that contains zinc. Dr. Shippen recommends 50 mgs twice a day until you see improvement and then 50 mgs after that.[5]
• Lose weight. Enough said.
• Cut down on any heavy alcohol use. Alcohol's beneficial effects can be obtained through as little as one to three servings per week.
• If you're taking diuretics for high blood pressure, increase your zinc supplementation to compensate.
• Look for organically grown produce and watch your exposure to environmental chemicals. You're already producing plenty of estrogen; you don't need to go looking for estrogen-mimicking imposters!

WEEK 8 🦋 DAY 5

Today's Thin Thought: Take time each day to care for yourself.

Your daily assignments:
  • **Drink lots of water.**

5. Ibid, page 191.

- Bend, stretch, and use your weights upon waking.
- Walk in the morning for at least thirty minutes.
- Keep track of what you put in your mouth.
- Watch your servings/portions.
- Watch your intake of unhealthy fats.
- Move more during the day.
- Choose a variety of whole foods over fragmented foods.
- Take a good multivitamin/multimineral.
- Enhance your diet with nutritional supplements.
- Intentionally pursue a good night's sleep.

SETTING THE DAY FOR SUCCESS

Allow me to speak to the women for a moment today. In the past, many women dealt with menopausal symptoms by utilizing hormone replacement therapy (HRT). As an additional benefit, it was thought HRT would help women cut down on coronary heart disease and osteoporosis. Recently, the Women's Health Initiative trial that looked at HRT using estrogen and progestin (a synthetic form of progesterone) was curtailed after preliminary results showed an increase in cancer risk and heart disease.[6] (The part of the trial studying supplementation of estrogen alone is continuing and is slated to be completed in 2005.)

In Seattle, Dr. Garnet I. Anderson at the Fred Hutchison Cancer Research Center has found that the risks for ovarian cancer in women on hormone re-

6. Cauley, Jane A., et al., "Effects of Estrogen Plus Progestin on Risk of Fracture and Bone Mineral Density: The Women's Health Initiative Randomized Trial, *Journal of the American Medical Association* 290 (2003): 1729–1738.

placement therapy outweighed any benefits from lower risks of womb or endometrial cancer. In addition, over the past several years, other risks have come to light, including an increase in invasive breast cancer,[7] a rare form of breast cancer,[8] coronary heart disease, stroke, and pulmonary embolism,[9] and double the risk of dementia, including Alzheimer's, in women over sixty-five.[10] These were all in trials with a combination of estrogen and progesterone or progestin. These studies certainly warrant caution in hormone replacement therapy for healthy menopausal women with a uterus.

But what can be done for women who are experiencing the uncomfortable and sometimes debilitating effects of menopause? I believe the answer lies in the use of hormonal transdermal creams. Essentially,

7. http://www.fhcrc.org/news/science/2003/06/24/hrt.html. Website is for the Fred Hutchison Cancer Research Center. Name of press release is "Long-Term Use of Combined Hormone-Replacement Therapy Poses Significant Breast-Cancer Risk, Regardless of Regimen."

8. http://www.fhcrc.og/news/science/2000/05/1/hormone.html. Website is for the Fred Hutchison Cancer Research Center. Name of press release is "Combined Hormone-Replacement Therapy May Boost Incidence of Rare Form of Breast Cancer."

9. www.fhcrc.org/pubs/center_news/2002/jul18/sart1.html. Website is for the Fred Hutchison Cancer Research Center. Name of science article is "Early end for HRT clinical trial: Combination of estrogen and progestin proves more risky than healthful, triggering halt of first definitive, large, national study of hormone therapy." Release date is July 18, 2002. Author is Barbara Berg.

10. www.fhcrc.org/pubs/center_news/2003/jun19/sart2.html. Website is for the Fred Hutchison Cancer Research Center. Name of science article is "Combined hormone-replacement therapy: Risk of dementia adds to list of concerns. After linking estrogen plus progestin to increased risk of breast cancer, heart disease and stroke, Women's Health Initiative researchers discover cognitive connection." Release date is June 19, 2003. Author is Barbara Berg.

these are creams rubbed on the body that contain natural estrogens from plants such as wild yam extract. The hormones in these creams are in much smaller concentrations than those used in HRT and are absorbed through the skin. There are versions with estrogen only, or with a mixture of estrogen and progesterone.

I have found them to be amazingly helpful for women who experience severe symptoms and wish to avoid the risks involved in traditional hormone replacement therapy.

While the bad news on HRT seems to pop up in the media on a regular basis, the good news is that transdermal creams are a wonderful alternative. I encourage you to investigate whether these might be of benefit to you. Talk to your physician or health care professional about transdermal creams.

SUCCESS IN ACTION

It can seem that, as a woman, you are always having to make adjustments for the hormonal fluctuations of your body. First it was puberty, then before, during and after each menstrual cycle, then any pregnancies that came along, now perimenopause, menopause, and postmenopause. Through all of this, some women come to hate and distrust their bodies. How do you really feel about your body as a woman? I'd like you to go back and think about your relationship with your body over the course of your life. How do you feel about it now, today? Is it time you made peace with your body? It is not your enemy. It is not somehow flawed because of the hormonal ebbs and tides hardwired into it. Rather, the female body is an extraordinarily complex entity with astonishing strength, flexibility, and stamina. If you have not done so before, it's time to celebrate your female body! Many women find their postmenopausal years to be a time of grace, maturity, emotional steadiness, peace, and calm. This is the wonderful future ahead, when you listen to your body and adjust and adapt instead of agitate.

WEEK 8   🦋   DAY 6

Today's Thin Thought: Maturing as a man means more than machismo.

Your daily assignments:
- **Drink lots of water.**
- **Bend, stretch, and use your weights upon waking.**
- **Walk in the morning for at least thirty minutes.**
- **Keep track of what you put in your mouth.**
- **Watch your servings/portions.**
- **Watch your intake of unhealthy fats.**
- **Move more during the day.**
- **Choose a variety of whole foods over fragmented foods.**
- **Take a good multivitamin/multimineral.**
- **Enhance your diet with nutritional supplements.**
- **Intentionally pursue a good night's sleep.**

SETTING THE DAY FOR SUCCESS

Today I'd like to focus primarily on you men. We've already talked about the importance of keeping off excess weight, taking supplements, especially zinc, and maintaining a healthy sex life as ways to support your body's production of testosterone. Testosterone is not only used in sexual functioning, it also gives you your can-do attitude and zest for life.

It makes you more positive, energetic, and optimistic. By keeping your weight down and your percentage of lean muscle up, you're not just going to feel better about how your body looks, you're going to feel better about yourself—period.

There is another way you can help yourself look and feel better (and it works well for women, too). It's through supplementation with a compound called dehydroepiandrosterone (DHEA). Produced in the adrenal gland, this steroid hormone is found in sexes. The body takes DHEA and turns it into a variety of hormones. When testosterone declines, so does DHEA. When DHEA levels in older adults are returned to levels found in younger people, they feel better physically and mentally. In a clinical trial with men and women aged forty to seventy, participants were given 50 mgs. of DHEA every night for six months (in a placebo-based, randomized study). Those who took the DHEA were found to have improvements in mental functioning such as mood and stress, as well as physical improvements such as energy level and sleep quality.[11]

DHEA is a supplement that can be found in most major health, nutrition, or supplement stores. Skeptical? Why not try this out and see if it doesn't cause an improvement for you? So much of *Thin over 40* is about feeling good about yourself and your future. Concerned about taking a "foreign" substance? Think of it as giving back to your body what it naturally had when you were younger.

11. Morales A. J., et al. "Effects of Replacement Dose of DHEA in Men and Women of Advancing Age. *J Clin Endo Metab* 76, no. 6 (1944): 1360–1367, as referenced in "Male Menopause" by Edward D. Rosick, *Life Extention* magazine, October 2003, pages 71–71.

SUCCESS IN ACTION

It has been my experience, working with both men and women over the years on health and weight issues, that women are more amenable to seeking professional help for how they feel, be it a physician, nutritionist, or counselor. Men can be reluctant to go to someone for help. I ascribe it to a natural reluctance to (a) admit anything is wrong, and (b) submit to the expertise or authority of another person. In your journal today, I'd like you to think about your interactions with others regarding your weight and health. This could be your spouse, friends, acquaintances, or health care professionals. If you chafe at the idea of having to go to the doctor or resent your wife lecturing you about a nutritional supplement she thinks you should take, think about why that is. What negatives do you associate with it? Are those realistic or do they come from a fear or aversion from your past? Be honest with your answers.

Let's face it: As we age we need to establish positive, supportive relationships with our health care providers. They can be important sources of information, help, and encouragement in our *Thin over 40* goals. If the whole of idea of taking pills or going to the doctor is onerous to you, you need to investigate why and jettison any outdated, misguided notions that could keep you from obtaining the support these important professionals can play in your life.

WEEK 8   🦋   DAY 7

Today's Thin Thought: You can help out your hormones by what you eat.

Your daily assignments:
• **Drink lots of water.**

- Bend, stretch, and use your weights upon waking.
- Walk in the morning for at least thirty minutes.
- Keep track of what you put in your mouth.
- Watch your servings/portions.
- Watch your intake of unhealthy fats.
- Move more during the day.
- Choose a variety of whole foods over fragmented foods.
- Take a good multivitamin/multimineral.
- Enhance your diet with nutritional supplements.
- Intentionally pursue a good night's sleep.

Weekly Assignment:
- Go grocery shopping for next week.

SETTING THE DAY FOR SUCCESS

Because this is the day you go grocery shopping for the week, it's the perfect day for you to recommit to eating a healthy diet. And by healthy, I want to stress a well-balanced diet that includes lots of fruits and vegetables, healthy fats, lean protein and proper water intake. These are all important to *Thin over 40* and they have the added bonus of being extremely beneficial for you as you go through menopause or andropause. There is a hormonal tectonic shift going on in your body and it needs all of the vitamins, minerals, and nutrients it can get to help accomplish this process.

- *Fresh vegetables and fruit*. This is important to both genders. Whenever possible, look for organically grown produce. Many people are chemically sensitive to pesticides. In addition, one study has shown a link between the pesticide compound methoxychlor and a decrease in testosterone production because of its estrogenlike properties.[12] Women should eat at least five servings per day, especially of green, leafy vegetables, which are rich in nutrients and phytochemicals. Phytochemicals include phytoestrogens, which are estrogen compounds found in plants, especially in soybeans and flaxseed. These can help augment low estrogen during menopause.

- *Lean meats.* Protein is important in the production of muscle tissue. Men, lean muscle is a component of testosterone production, so the less muscle you have, the more your testosterone production is compromised. Women, you also need to be sure to eat protein in order to assist in muscle protection. Lean beef is fine, but remember that poultry has a higher protein content than beef. Pork is also an excellent choice for a lean, white meat. Women need to be sure that they do not eat too much protein. Calcium, a necessary component in bone production, can be compromised by too much protein, increasing the risk of loss of bone density and osteoporosis.

- *Fish.* We've talked about the benefits of fish before because of the omega-3 oils they contain. These oils can help women alleviate vaginal dryness. For men, the fatty acids found in fish, EPH and DHA, are also extremely beneficial, as they reduce cholesterol levels and can help thwart the production

---

12. Akingbemi, B. T., et al. "A metabolite of Methoxychlor Reduces Testosterone Biosynthesis." *Population Briefs, Population Council* 5, no. 4 (1999): 31–32, as referenced in "Male Menopause" by Edward D. Rosick, *Life Extension* magazine, October 2003, page 69.

of a compound that binds up free testosterone in a man's system, leaving less available testosterone.

- *Water.* I can't stress enough the importance of water, especially in the area of fat metabolism. Water lubricates life and acts as a transport vehicle for many bodily functions, not the least of which is toxin removal. During menopause, women can become more dehydrated, so make sure to drink your water! Water also helps flush out toxins produced by the breakdown of muscle tissue you experience when you exercise. Sweat uses up even more water, so increase your water intake to compensate for your increased activity level.

SUCCESS IN ACTION

As you make up your shopping list today, take time to jot down how each of these items is going to help your body with the transition through menopause or andropause. If you have already gone through this change, write down how each item is going to bring you closer to the vitality and health you desire. As you put each item in your cart this week, visualize it inside your body. Envision how it will help your *Thin Over 40* goals. Remember, there are no totally evil foods, when consumed in moderation. If you want to purchase some ice cream, at least it has calcium. Even chocolate mimics endorphins. Be wise, but don't be rigid. Rigidity leads to failure. This isn't a diet, it's a way of life.

HERO OF THE WEEK

As we end this week, I'd like to introduce you to Dee. After the birth of her second child, Dee came to realize "something was wrong." She didn't feel like herself. She was tired and cranky all of the time. Her fatigue and lethargy got worse and worse, until depression set in. Her physician put her on Zoloft, and later Prozac which helped for a while. But over the years, Dee began to hear more and more media reports about people experiencing negative side effects of taking Prozac. She became nervous and uncomfortable taking it. Dee didn't want to return to those dark days when she could barely function and each day was a struggle. She was afraid of continuing to take Prozac and afraid of what she might become if she didn't.

I suggested she begin using one of the transdermal creams, ProFeminell. Within four months, Dee was off Prozac, saying, "I didn't need it anymore. The ProFeminell cream made that possible. I've been using the cream for about three years now. I call it my Happy Cream!"

At fifty-one years old, Dee is navigating menopause with a minimum of unpleasant symptoms, including the absence of hot flashes. She's supporting her body naturally and her optimism and outlook on life and the future have never been better! Dee, thank you for being our Hero of the Week!

Week 9
Making the Most of Balance

Week 9 ❦ Day 1

Today's Thin Thought: Binge eating is controlled eating.

Welcome to the new week! You've successfully navigated two months of *Thin over 40* and are preparing to launch into your third! This week we're going to be talking about why people engage in what some have characterized as out-of-control eating. This binge eating can sabotage your *Thin over 40* lifestyle and produce copious amounts of frustration, as well as excess weight. It's the time you eat half a quart of ice cream or half a bag of cookies. It's when you sit down to eat a light supper and end up consuming that plus all the leftovers in the refrigerator. It's called a binge because you're eating more than is necessary to create physical fullness. You feel compelled to eat this way, but are your binges really out of control? Or do they represent a time when you are very much in control, but choosing to engage in a behavior that is counterproductive to being *Thin over 40?* Are there other times when you seem to have a craving, a physical imperative, to eat a certain way, even when you know it's not good for you? That's what we're going to be talking about this week.

Our Key Concept for the week is Balance. Binge

eating is the bane of balance. Throughout this week we're going to look at what causes binge behavior and what you can do to take positive steps to reintroduce balance into the way you approach food and eating. Each day, we'll highlight a different challenge and present suggestions for meeting and overcoming that challenge.

Your daily assignments:
(Are you getting tired of seeing these each day? Have you gotten to the point where your eyes just skim over them, without really looking? If so, this week, I want you to focus each day on really reading over, and agreeing with, this list. You must own it and internalize it! The reason for seeing these every single day is to have them so ingrained in your mind they become part of your internal dialogue. So that, for example, by midmorning you realize you haven't had enough water. Or, when reaching for that doughnut or pastry you remember that you are watching your intake of bad fats. Or, before leaving for work, you are prompted to take your supplements for the day. We're going over and over these so they become your marching orders for each day, as you journey step-by-step to *Thin over 40* success.)

- **Drink lots of water.** So important with your increased activity levels.
- **Bend, stretch, and use your weights upon waking.** Doesn't it feel great to help prepare your body for your day?
- **Walk for at least thirty-five minutes today.** As we increase the amount of walking time, it's fine to break this up over the course of the day. A caution, however: I always do the bulk of my exercise in the morning before I start my day.

Otherwise, the normal pressures of the day can crowd out this important daily routine. I make it a priority by making it first.

- **Keep track of what you put in your mouth.** That's really what this week is going to focus on—what you put in your mouth and why.
- **Watch your servings/portions.**
- **Watch your intake of unhealthy fats.**
- **Move more during the day.**
- **Choose a variety of whole foods over fragmented foods.**
- **Take a good multivitamin/multimineral.**
- **Enhance your diet with nutritional supplements.**
- **Intentionally pursue a good night's sleep.**
- **Strategically combat your cravings.** Now, aren't you glad you didn't miss this one! For many of you, this point is crucial to your success.

SETTING THE DAY FOR SUCCESS

Do you binge eat? In other words, are there times when you just feel like eating but aren't really hungry? Is it triggered by feelings of frustration, stress, loneliness? *Thin over 40* eating is balanced eating. So if there are times when your eating is unbalanced, it's time to take a look at why.

There is a recognized mental disorder known as binge-eating disorder. It is characterized by eating very rapidly, eating beyond full to uncomfortable, eating large amounts of food even when not hungry, eating alone out of embarrassment or shame, and after bingeing, feeling ashamed, disgusted, depressed, or guilty. I'm not suggesting you have this diagnosable disorder, but within that definition are the seeds of disordered eating, even if it's not an eating disorder. I would like you to consider those times when you eat even when not feeling hungry. I would like you to examine what you eat during those times and why you choose to eat this way.

I know that some of you may be chaffing at the word "choose." Let me explain why I use that. In my work with eating disorders, I have found that eating disorder behavior begins as a choice. The person makes a conscious decision to begin to respond to food a certain way. Over the course of the disorder, its progressive nature leads to compulsion, but at the onset, there is choice. Many will use food as an acceptable form of rebellion and comfort. It may stem from childhood, where there was constant pressure to eat everything on their plate—and they responded by restricting food. Others come from a home environment where physical perfection is emphasized to such a degree, they binge as a way to numb their feelings of insecurity and lack of acceptance, and purge in order to "undo the damage" and avoid unwanted weight gain.

I also see people who have, over the years, turned to food as a way to deal with uncomfortable feelings of sadness, disappointment, or frustration. These people also express a certain rebellion through food against all of the pressures they feel in life. They may feel powerless over that dead-end job or loveless marriage or contentious relationship with their children, but there is one thing about their life they can control—their food choices. Over the years, they have turned to comfort foods as a way to gain back a small measure of personal control. They figure, if life doesn't feel good, food certainly does. They also rebel against age. Tired of wishing for a body they feel they can no longer have, they fight back by giving in. Food is used as a form of control, but it does nothing to deal with the real issues—it doesn't give any lasting relief and, by eating the wrong types of foods, it robs the person of the ability to generate the physical stamina necessary for optimism, hope, and joy. In short, as they age they become larger and more depressed. It's time to stop this cycle and take charge! If this pattern speaks to you, realize you've already made significant improvements by adopting what you're learning through *Thin over 40*. You're ready to tackle the stubborn issue of binge eating.

SUCCESS IN ACTION

You've been journaling what you eat every day since you began this program. I want you to be honest about something—have you written down accurately when you've binged? When you've eaten half a bag of chips or a quart of ice cream? Did you dutifully factor how many calories you'd just taken in? Or did you leave that off, while promising yourself you wouldn't do it again so it didn't really count?

If you have been writing these down, go back over your journal and look for patterns of location, time of day, and choice of binge foods. Even if you haven't been writing them down, you still know what they are. Most people have a list of binge foods and even times when they feel justified to binge. Bad day. PMS. Fight with the (boss, kids, spouse—you fill in the blank). Watching a movie. Your job today is to identify where, when, and what. We'll continue to work through the why.

WEEK 9 🦋 DAY 2

Today's Thin Thought: Problems are not solved by putting something in your mouth.

Your daily assignments:
• **Drink lots of water.**

- Bend, stretch, and use your weights upon waking.
- Walk for at least thirty-five minutes today.
- Keep track of what you put in your mouth.
- Watch your servings/portions.
- Watch your intake of unhealthy fats.
- Move more during the day.
- Choose a variety of whole foods over fragmented foods.
- Take a good multivitamin/multimineral.
- Enhance your diet with nutritional supplements.
- Intentionally pursue a good night's sleep.
- Strategically combat your cravings.

SETTING THE DAY FOR SUCCESS

Today, let's look at the "when" part of the binge equation. You'll find there are certain times you eat too much. Daily life and full schedules are highly stressful and you can be fooled by the body into thinking what you need is a caloric pick-me-up. Snack food advertisers promote certain high-calorie, high-fat foods like candy bars as a way to make it through the afternoon. We're used to responding to our body's low time by giving it something to eat. The real reason for that dip in energy doesn't matter. We respond by popping something into our mouths. Feel tired—pop. Feel anxious—pop. Feel frustrated—pop. Feel tense—pop. Feel cranky—pop. Feel bored—pop.

Here are some other times you want to be aware of:

- *Mornings, right upon waking.* We've talked about using a high-caffeine and/or high-calorie infusion to jump-start the day.

- *Midmorning or midafternoon.* This could be nothing more than the stress involved in waiting either for that lunch break or end of the day. Your body may be asking for you to get up and relieve the stress. You suddenly feel a drop in energy or a need for a diversion from what you're doing. It's easy and convenient to provide that break through food. Even when a snack is the appropriate response, our choice of what that snack is can be inappropriate.
- *At night after the evening meal.* Many people give themselves "permission" to relax only after they've gotten everything done or are too tired to care anymore. Evening then becomes a time to let down, to relax. And relaxing has come to mean eating or snacking, often something salty or sweet. It's the bag of chips while the game's on or the pound cake during a favorite drama. You're not hungry, you're keyed up; and the way you've chosen to calm down is through food.

SUCCESS IN ACTION

I want you to look at the patterns to your binge or nonhunger eating. Recognize they're not due to hunger but are how you cope with physical or emotional discomfort. For example, upon waking, your body is gearing up by increasing metabolism, heart rate, and blood pressure. This is perfectly normal, but it can leave you feeling a little fuzzy as you adjust. Check to make sure you're still drinking your water right upon waking. Rehydrating after sleep can help regulate your blood pressure. The physical activity you're doing in the morning helps clear out the mental cobwebs. Use your body's own stimulants to get you going instead of caffeine.

For those midmorning or midafternoon times, get up and move around. You needn't interpret every sign of physical sluggishness as a need to pop something into your mouth. Stretch, move around, get some fresh air—these are all nonfood alternatives.

Night eating can be the stumbling block for many. We push and prod ourselves during the day. We don't get enough sleep. We have far too much stress. Evening comes, the sun sets, and we want to eat for comfort. After the noise of the day, the quiet of the evening allows the echo of loneliness, frustration, or distress to be heard, prompting a reach for food to comfort.

Whatever the reason, too many of us think getting ready for bed means filling up our stomachs. Working through this entrenched pattern may mean you need to stop eating in the evening, after dinner, completely. As an alcoholic must abstain from alcohol, if you are prone to night eating, you need to remove snacking after dinner as an activity. The goal is to go to bed with your stomach mostly cleared out from dinner. It needs a rest overnight, too. What you don't need are those digesting calories turning to fat while you sleep!

WEEK 9 🦋 DAY 3

Today's Thin Thought: Your stomach may be full while your heart is hungry.

Your daily assignments:
- **Drink lots of water.**
- **Bend, stretch, and use your weights upon waking.**
- **Walk for at least thirty-five minutes today.**
- **Keep track of what you put in your mouth.**
- **Watch your servings/portions.**

- Watch your intake of unhealthy fats.
- Move more during the day.
- Choose a variety of whole foods over fragmented foods.
- Take a good multivitamin/multimineral.
- Enhance your diet with nutritional supplements.
- Intentionally pursue a good night's sleep.
- Strategically combat your cravings.

Your weekly assignment:
- Weigh yourself.

SETTING THE DAY FOR SUCCESS

Bingeing is not merely a desire for a candy bar or a jar of peanuts that overtakes you. It's not just grabbing a handful of cookies when you get home from work as you're preparing dinner. Rather, it's an intense, focused desire to practically shove food into your mouth. It has nothing to do with physical hunger and everything to do with emotional hunger. This emotional feeling, however, is so strong, it can be interpreted as physical. Physical or emotional? Sometimes it's hard to know the difference.

Generally, physical hunger can wait a bit. It's there, it's noticeable, but you can hold off. Generally, that warning, that burning in your stomach will go away if you ignore it. Oh, it will return, but not right away, especially if you're engaged in some interesting activity. When your stomach starts to rumble, then you know you're pushing the limit because your gastric juices are complaining. That's physical hunger, and it comes on gradually, as your stores of food are utilized by the body and it lets you know it's ready for more. Physical hunger can usually be ignored for a while.

Emotional hunger can be identified by its sudden appearance, by its susceptibility to outside stimuli, and by its compelling nature. Like the hit of a fish on a pole, emotional hunger can strike without warning. Detached from a physical imperative, the subconscious is free to demand satisfaction from food at any moment. You may have been mulling over how that offhand comment yesterday made you feel. Resentful and bitter, the impulse strikes to throw caution to the wind and immediately overeat. And I do mean immediately. One of the signposts of emotional eating is that it's imperative. Once you've decided the only way to feel better is to eat, few things are allowed to come between you and food. You'll go out of your way to get exactly what you want.

Catching the glimpse or a whiff of a favorite food can also produce an emotional eating response. Your sense of smell has powerful ties to your emotions. Smells can provoke an amazing emotional connection to memories and associations. You may not be remotely hungry when you catch the mouthwatering odor of buttered popcorn or a fresh-baked pastry. All at once, you have to have it. Again, the imperative. It's about self-gratification, not hunger.

Most of us in this country never go long enough between eating to produce the kind of physical need that emotional eating counterfeits. It feels like we're starving but deep down we know we're not. The desire for relief from that feeling of emptiness, of deprivation, is so great, however, we obey.

I completely agree that we should give our bodies what we need. What I disagree on is that something is always food. I agree we feel a lack, or loss, emotionally, and that needs to be addressed. But instead of always defaulting to food, we need to take time to evaluate the source of the true hunger and then find a way to fill it that doesn't involve empty promises through empty calories.

SUCCESS IN ACTION

When we fill up that emotional need with food, we never take the time to really meditate on the true source of our hunger. Food is much more convenient. Food feels better. Often, this hunger is one we've lived with for years, and we simply would rather drown our sorrows in food than truly experience it and deal with it, in order to flush it from our systems.

I want you to think about the times you eat emotionally. What feelings trigger this overwhelming desire? Is it loneliness? Is it anger or resentment? Is it grief? Food, being so abundant in our society, is a convenient, legal form of self-medication. But it just masks the symptoms; it doesn't get at the root of the pain.

Spend some time with your journal today, thinking about the types of pain you find yourself self-medicating through food. Make a list. Now, think back to the time or times in your life when you first remember feeling that pain. Ask yourself if the pain you've identified today has gotten tied into that pain from the past.

Forty-plus years is a long time to be carrying around this kind of pain. If you've identified some deeply rooted pain from your past, I encourage you to talk to someone about it. Depending upon the type of pain, speaking to a family member or a friend can provide needed relief. I cannot tell you the number of times I've sat in my office and listened to someone open up for the first time, after years of living in pain. I've seen people who have padded the pain of rejection, abuse, abandonment, cruelty, or neglect

with pounds and pounds of fat by trying to stuff it
farther and farther away with food. Please believe
me when I say this never works. Only by understanding and releasing the pain will it ever go away.
If you cannot do this through family, friends, or faith
community, please seek professional help today.
Emotional eating can point directly to an unresolved
hurt in your life. Isn't it time to do what you need
to heal?

WEEK 9   🦋   DAY 4

Today's Thin Thought: Liquor may be quicker,
but candy's still dandy.

Your daily assignments:
- **Drink lots of water.**
- **Bend, stretch, and use your weights upon
  waking.**
- **Walk for at least thirty-five minutes today.**
- **Keep track of what you put in your mouth.**
- **Watch your servings/portions.**
- **Watch your intake of unhealthy fats.**
- **Move more during the day.**
- **Choose a variety of whole foods over frag-
  mented foods.**
- **Take a good multivitamin/multimineral.**
- **Enhance your diet with nutritional supple-
  ments.**
- **Intentionally pursue a good night's sleep.**
- **Strategically combat your cravings.**

SETTING THE DAY FOR SUCCESS

Recently, I read a fascinating item in a fitness magazine. It talked about a study done at the University
of Wisconsin, where rats were fed a high-fat, high-

sugar, high-salt diet. Of course, the rats didn't have any choice; they could eat only what they were given. An interesting thing happened, though, when the rats were returned to a healthy diet. They developed symptoms consistent with withdrawal. The lead researcher, Dr. Matthew Will, believes the high-fat, -sugar, and -salt diet altered the rats' brain biochemistry "with effects similar to those of powerful opiates such as morphine."[1] Simply put, the rats got "hooked" on the bad food to the point of a physical alteration in their brain chemistry.

As we look at why we eat certain foods in inappropriate quantities, we need to be open to the possibility that when we say chocolate is our "nightly fix," we're not just engaging in harmless hyperbole. Still think this is far-fetched? It isn't to Princeton University's Bart Hoebel, who in 2002 released the results of his own study with rats. The rats were made to binge on sugar. Then the effects of the sugar were blocked. At that point, the rats experienced withdrawal symptoms such as "the shakes" and brain chemistry changes, linked to sugar's ability to stimulate the brain's own opiates. Hoebel said, "The brain is getting addicted to its own opioids as it would to morphine or heroin. Drugs give a bigger effect, but it is essentially the same process."[2] You choose these foods for a reason—they stimulate the pleasure center of the brain. Sugar consumption, and its effect, can produce a druglike response. And we eat a lot of sugar every day, every year.

For you to have long-term success in your *Thin*

1. No authors listed. "Nutrition Spotlight: Edible Essentials," *ACE Fitness Matters* magazine, Vol. 8, Issue 5, page 6.
2. Hoebel, Bart. http://www.princeton.edu/pr/news/02/q2/0620-hoebel.htm. "Sugar on the Brain: Study Shows Sugar Dependence in Rats," June 20, 2002.

over 40 lifestyle, you need to cut down on your consumption of sugar. This may prove extremely difficult if you have developed an addictive reaction to sugar. Simply put, for a while you may not feel the best. Cravings, headaches, muscle tension, and irritability are all symptoms of withdrawal—just ask anyone who has tried to quit smoking.

At The Center, we've helped many individuals "come down" off sugar, as they work to incorporate healthier eating. It isn't easy at first, but after making it through the withdrawal symptoms, they report feeling better and losing weight. We encourage them to avoid as much processed sugar as possible and choose fruits as a sweet alternative. Another interesting effect has been reported—when they return to eating some sugar, they say they feel satisfied with a much smaller amount. In fact, if they eat "too much" sugar, they experience nausea and headaches. They have learned that a little bit of sugar goes a long way.

SUCCESS IN ACTION

Look back and reflect on how much, and how many times, you reach for sugar during the day. Write down your favorite sweet foods. How many times a day do you eat them? Do you find yourself "unable to stop?" Are you able to eat one piece of candy? A few M&M's? One scoop of ice cream? There is nothing wrong with some sugar in your diet, but it should come through fruits, starches, and complex carbohydrates, as opposed to processed sugar. See if you are able to go the rest of today without eating any sweets. Note how many times you experienced a craving. Tell yourself you don't need to eat sweets today. Write down how you are feeling and make sure to drink lots of water.

WEEK 9 🦋 DAY 5

Today's Thin Thought: Some cravings are physical in nature.

Your daily assignments:
- **Drink lots of water.**
- **Bend, stretch, and use your weights upon waking.**
- **Walk for at least thirty-five minutes today.**
- **Keep track of what you put in your mouth.**
- **Watch your servings/portions.**
- **Watch your intake of unhealthy fats.**
- **Move more during the day.**
- **Choose a variety of whole foods over fragmented foods.**
- **Take a good multivitamin/multimineral.**
- **Enhance your diet with nutritional supplements.**
- **Intentionally pursue a good night's sleep.**
- **Strategically combat your cravings.**

SETTING THE DAY FOR SUCCESS

I hope yesterday went well and you were able to make it through the day without eating any processed sugar. I'd like you to try it again today and see how you feel. For some of you, it may be a matter of retooling an established habit. For others, this drop in sugar consumption may have set off a major craving. The culprit could be a compromised digestive system, not a lack of willpower. Over the years, I've seen firsthand the effects of a small, simple-celled organism called *Candida albans,* or yeast. A vast majority of those I've treated with eating disorders have an overgrowth of yeast in their systems. Eating disorders can produce yeast blooms in the body and so can other more common conditions, such as medication and antibiotic use, or simply poor nutritional habits.

While many of you may be unfamiliar with candida, most of you are aware of yeast. When used in breads, yeast is combined with three things—heat, moisture, and sugar—to grow. It's no different for your body. Yeast loves to find moist, warm areas. In the nose and mouth, a yeast overgrowth is called thrush. But yeast can grow just about anywhere. It is especially fond of the intestinal tract and the vagina. This is why women can be plagued with recurrent yeast infections.

Everyone has yeast colonies inside, which are kept in check by healthy digestive bacteria. These healthy bacteria can be decimated, however, by the stress of a chronic illness or simply a prolonged exposure to stress, antibiotics, or certain medications. When the healthy bacteria are compromised, yeast flourishes. Yeast, being simple, demands only one thing really— sugar. The more candida in the system, the more intense cravings can be for sugary foods. (For a greater look at the role of yeast in a variety of conditions, I recommend you read Dr. William Crook's book entitled, *The Yeast Connection*.[3] Dr. Crook has done much of the pioneering work on this subject, which has yet to receive total support in the medical community at large. I believe in his work because I have seen the devastation caused by yeast overgrowth for twenty years.)

SUCCESS IN ACTION

Continue to monitor how you are feeling this week as you seek to reduce or eliminate the amount of

3. Crook, William G. *The Yeast Connection: A Medical Breakthrough.* New York: Vintage, 1986.

processed sugars you eat. If you have a concern about the intensity of cravings and suspect a yeast connection, I encourage you to obtain a copy of Dr. Crook's book. In addition, a simple stool test can determine the level of candida in your system. (Again, not all physicians make a correlation between the presence of yeast and sugar cravings.)

There are a couple of things you can do to help support digestive health. You're already doing the first by eating healthier. You can also look for products with *acidophilus* and *bifidus* added. These are healthy digestive bacteria and are often found in milk products (look on the label to make sure they have been added) and to yogurt (the label should say that it comes with active cultures). In addition, you can take extra acidophilus and bifidus by capsule. Adding healthy bacteria to your digestive tract is highly beneficial. In addition, to help control an existing yeast overgrowth, we have developed a product at The Center called Canditrol, which inhibits yeast growth. (For more information about these products, please go to www.thinover40.com or call our toll-free number: 888-771-5166.)

WEEK 9 🦋 DAY 6

Today's Thin Thought: We often crave what we should avoid.

Your daily assignments:
- **Drink lots of water.**
- **Bend, stretch, and use your weights upon waking.**
- **Walk for at least thirty-five minutes today.**
- **Keep track of what you put in your mouth.**
- **Watch your servings/portions.**
- **Watch your intake of unhealthy fats.**

- Move more during the day.
- Choose a variety of whole foods over fragmented foods.
- Take a good multivitamin/multimineral.
- Enhance your diet with nutritional supplements.
- Intentionally pursue a good night's sleep.
- Strategically combat your cravings.

SETTING THE DAY FOR SUCCESS

Today we're going to look at another reason for food cravings. It's true that we often crave the very things that aren't good for us. This is certainly true in the area of food sensitivities. Let me take a minute to differentiate food sensitivities from food allergies. Food allergies cause a specific response from your immune system and create a range of symptoms from a tingly mouth, to hives, to life-threatening anaphylactic shock.

Food sensitivities can come about when you do not introduce variety into your diet. In other words, if you eat the same type of food over and over, you can develop sensitivity to it. The most common sensitivities are to wheat, eggs, and dairy products. Problems can also develop if your intestinal tract is not properly digesting your food. Poorly digested food particles enter the bloodstream and your organs. Your body responds to this irritation in a perfectly understandable way—it causes inflammation in an effort to cushion the effects. This inflammation is handled through water retention. Like a blister that forms when you injure your big toe, the body uses water to cushion the site of the irritant. The result is you feel bloated and uncomfortable.

When your body has developed a food sensitivity,

it can actually crave the food that caused it, experiencing withdrawal symptoms of fatigue, headaches, fibromyalgia, and irritability. With wheat sensitivities, people experience intense cravings for wheat products like bread. After ingesting the wheat product, they experience a temporary respite from the symptoms. Of course, the symptoms return because wheat's been eaten. The symptoms return as does the desire to eat the product again to mitigate those symptoms. Over and over it goes.

About the only way to determine if you've developed sensitivity to a certain food is to temporarily remove it from your diet. While wheat is the most common sensitivity I've found because of how pervasive it is in foods, it is possible to remove or reduce the amount of wheat ingested. It takes some investigation of other sources of flour, such as rye, barley, and oat. As in the case of sugar, by cutting back on your consumption you may first experience some discomfort, but those feelings should fade and you'll actually start to feel much better. Once you've cleansed the food item from your diet, you can choose to use alternatives or begin to slowly reintroduce small amounts. You can also obtain the help of a health care professional to investigate whether you have an allergy to a specific food that could be causing some of your symptoms. An allergist can test you for a variety of common irritants, including different foods, and determine whether you should avoid any specific food.

SUCCESS IN ACTION

Look over the foods you predominantly eat, especially breads and sweets. Sometimes it is difficult to tell whether you have developed an emotional attachment to them or a food sensitivity. I encourage you to seek the help of an allergist, nutritionist, or health care professional to determine if a food allergy or sensitivity is complicating your desire to be *Thin over 40*. There is help available! More and more professionals are recognizing this as a legitimate issue. By altering your food selection, and even increasing the variety of foods you eat, you can identify problem foods and make different choices.

Today, take a look at the top three foods you eat most frequently. Are they processed or whole, naturally sweet or sugared, naturally flavored or artificially salted? If your chosen three are processed, sugary, or salty, intentionally reduce your consumption. Pick healthier alternatives and give yourself permission to explore just how "hooked" you are to these foods.

WEEK 9　　🦋　　DAY 7

Today's Thin Thought: Make the most of your calories.

Your daily assignments:
- **Drink lots of water.**
- **Bend, stretch, and use your weights upon waking.**
- **Walk for at least thirty-five minutes today.**
- **Keep track of what you put in your mouth.**
- **Watch your servings/portions.**
- **Watch your intake of unhealthy fats.**
- **Move more during the day.**
- **Choose a variety of whole foods over fragmented foods.**
- **Take a good multivitamin/multimineral.**
- **Enhance your diet with nutritional supplements.**
- **Intentionally pursue a good night's sleep.**
- **Strategically combat your cravings.**

Weekly Assignment:
• **Go grocery shopping for next week.**

SETTING THE DAY FOR SUCCESS

Be proactive when you shop today and intentionally choose a wide variety of foods. Make sure they
are whole foods and reduce the number of processed
sweets. Your body needs specific nutrients to operate
this coming week. Give it healthy, revitalizing foods
and guard against the impulse to load your cart with
sugary or salty snacks. I won't argue that eating
those foods feels good, but so much of it is wasted
calories. Continue in your commitment to cut down
or eliminate sugar from your diet and journal how
you are feeling about and handling this decision.

You might want to consider making sure that the
multivitamin and mineral supplements you take
have biotin and chromium. Biotin helps regulate
blood sugar and can also be found in brewer's yeast,
cooked egg yolks, meat, milk, poultry, saltwater fish,
soybeans, and whole grains. The absorption of this
nutrient can be compromised by eating too many fats
and oils that have been heated up or exposed to air
for any length of time. Antibiotics, sulfa drugs, and
the artificial sweetener saccharin also interfere with
biotin.[4]

Chromium is needed for glucose metabolism and
helps maintain stable blood sugar levels by allowing
the body to utilize insulin. Diets high in "white
sugar, flour, and junk food" lead to a deficiency in
chromium.[5] It can be found in beer, brewer's yeast,

4. Balch, James F. M.D., and Phyllis A. Balch, C.N.C., *Prescription
   for Nutritional Healing: Second Edition.* Garden City Park, New
   York: Avery Publishing Group, 1997, page 17.
5. Ibid, page 24.

brown rice, cheese, meat, and whole grains. If you are diabetic and on insulin, you will need to consult your health care professional before taking supplemental chromium because it will alter your insulin requirements.

Another way you can help control sugar cravings is with L-Glutamine. Again, contact your health-care professional before taking L-Glutamine, as it is not for everyone. Those with kidney problems, Reye's syndrome, or any type of disorder that can result in an accumulation of ammonia in the blood should not take supplemental L-Glutamine.[6] But those who are able to take it should find a decrease in sugar cravings, as well as enhanced mental functioning.

SUCCESS IN ACTION

Many times, we are not aware of how sugar plays a role in both our positive and our negative moods. As you've been working toward reducing the amount, I'd like you to focus on how your body is feeling. Have you been successful warding off the cravings? Have you been able to substitute a glass of water, a piece of fruit, or a physical activity with success? Can you identify those cravings that are emotional in content (urgent, all-encompassing) from physical (that can be put off for a while)? Long-term success will require taming that sweet tooth, not only because of the calories involved but also the roller coaster of mind and body caused by fluctuating glucose and insulin levels. Dedicate yourself to this aspect of *Thin over 40* and I promise you, you'll feel great!

6. Ibid, page 39.

HERO OF THE WEEK

I am so pleased to be able to bring you this week's Hero because she is my wife, LaFon. While in college, after the death of her father, LaFon found herself turning increasingly to sweets for comfort. Though she had always been a thin person, she gained weight rapidly and felt terrible. She realized she was out of control and made a decision to choose only foods that didn't have obvious sugar in them. Instead of considering this a diet and a "negative," she chose to think of this as a positive way to return to feeling better and gaining control over her eating again. She didn't react in panic and starve herself, but, rather, over the course of two years, she lost the weight and established a healthy eating pattern that has served her well all of these years.

She says: Sugar no longer has power over my life choices. It doesn't even taste good to me anymore and a little goes a long way. In other words, my taste buds have adjusted and I simply don't want or feel a desire for as much of it. At age forty I'm in the best shape I've ever been in! What a blessing to know that food is not the boss of me—even if it gets the upper hand every once in a while!

LaFon is living with a healthy, realistic relationship to sugar, and she's feeling great. LaFon is my Hero of the Week.

WEEK 10
MAKING THE MOST OF RELATIONSHIPS

WEEK 10 🦋 DAY 1

Today's Thin Thought: People are a package deal; food is just packaged.

Ten weeks in! Allow me to say that you're amazing! You are focused and dedicated to your *Thin over 40* goal. Please continue with each aspect of the Plan as we gather momentum toward the last section of your training. And this is training because *Thin over 40* isn't a diet or an eating pattern for a set period of time; you're training for your new, healthy life. Keep with it. Internalize what you're learning and make it a part of you! It's about how you eat, but it's more about who you are and how you live.

So much of the time, we eat for reasons other than physical hunger. Because food is so readily available, we've used it as a cover for emotional distress brought on by feelings of anger, frustration, loneliness, sadness—anything that causes an emotional void. I've often found that the source of this void is pain from past relationships, unfulfilled present relationships, or the fear of future relationships. For this reason, the Key Concept for this tenth week is Relationships.

Each day this week, we're going to look at a different aspect of our relationships and determine if we have been using food as a way to cope. As long as these issues are left unresolved, the impetus to use food will continue. I cannot express to you the freedom that comes from successfully confronting damaging relationships and moving beyond them. By using food as a way to numb the negative feelings that arise from these relationships, we allow them to stay stuck where they are. Food cements the damaging effects of these negative relationships. *Thin over 40* is about unhooking yourself from these deadweights and surfacing to a happier, healthier life!

Your daily assignments: (Say them aloud to yourself each day. Listen to your voice and agree with yourself how important these are.)

- **Drink lots of water.** There's nothing as refreshing as a cool glass of water!
- **Bend, stretch, and use your weights upon waking.** Reach and stretch toward your goals!
- **Walk for at least forty minutes today.** Look forward to this time with joy! You're alive—you're moving—you're improving!
- **Keep track of what you put in your mouth.** Recognize each bite as nourishment and take the appropriate care with your body!
- **Watch your servings/portions.** You can do with less!
- **Watch your intake of unhealthy fats.** Visualize your arteries and organs.
- **Move more during the day.** Get up! Move around! Breathe deep!
- **Choose a variety of whole foods over fragmented foods.** Enjoy the crunch, taste, and texture of whole grains, fruits and vegetables!
- **Take a good multivitamin/multimineral.**
- **Enhance your diet with nutritional supplements.** Be wise and assist your body in ob-

taining the complex set of nutrients it needs to operate well!

- **Intentionally pursue a good night's sleep.** Give yourself permission to relax, rest, and sleep each night!
- **Strategically combat your cravings.** Be alert to whether it's your body or your mind doing the asking!
- **Cut down on processed sugars.** Allow your taste buds to adjust. You'll find that less really is more when it comes to sugar!

SETTING THE DAY FOR SUCCESS

Let's face it—people are messy. Even the happy ones get pouty. Even the mild-mannered ones get cranky. Even the most helpful say no. People are a mixed bag, a "package deal" of both good and bad. Food, on the other hand, has been packaged to look, smell, and taste appealing. The "good" is apparent and promoted; the "bad" is hidden on the back with small print and indecipherable labels. People are hard; food is easy. Is it any wonder, when relationships go bad, food looks so good?

It doesn't make it any easier when people and food are packaged together. Family mealtimes, holiday dinners, outing—all involve family, friends, and food. Is it any wonder that our relationship with food can become enmeshed in our relationships with other people? Of course not. But therein lies the challenge and the advantage of being over forty. It's a challenge because you've had more years to live and more relationships to become entangled with food. It's an advantage because, over forty, you have the maturity to understand how these relationships have become intertwined, and the wisdom to begin to unhook them.

Of all of your relationships—past, present, and future—I'd like to start by dealing with those in the past. It's been my experience that painful relationships from the past, often stemming from the family, are at the heart of many people's distorted connection with food. This connection to food develops because of the way food was presented within the family. For some, food was the universal pacifier in all situations, from revelry to distress. From ice cream when you were sick, to warm bread on rainy days after school, to pizza for celebrations, to "treats" on any sort of family errand or trip. Food was nourishment, yes, but it was also reward, comfort, and celebration.

For others, food was just nourishment. It was austere, colorless, unappealing. Food was presented as a necessary evil, to be consumed but rarely enjoyed. I've seen this to be true in homes where the mother suffered from an eating disorder of her own. The entire family was made to view food through her eyes—as the enemy. There was nothing relaxing about eating or food at home. *Away* from home was another matter entirely. Because of the austerity of food at home, the allure existed to enjoy food for pure pleasure away from home. As an adult—perpetually "away from home"—this can prove to be a problem. Understanding your background and how you grew up viewing food is essential. In order to do that, you need to examine those relationships, either in the past or ongoing, and begin to understand your feelings. Only then can you resist the pattern you've developed with food.

SUCCESS IN ACTION

Today, I want you to spend some time thinking about how your mother dealt with food. How did she deal with you? Do you remember being happy as a child? Was food a part of that happiness? Was there stress in your relationship with your mother growing up? How did you manage that stress as a child? Do you remember looking forward to certain foods or meals? What about other relationships in the family? Do you remember being able to express your feelings within the family? Do you remember sneaking or hiding food as a child? What were your favorite foods growing up? Do you still enjoy those today? What do you think of when you eat those foods? How do you feel?

If you overate as a child, what was the response? If your mother were standing right next to you as you overeat as an adult, what would her reaction be? How does that make you feel? Do you feel like an independent adult when you eat today? Or can you identify some lingering emotions from childhood creeping into your eating patterns? If you could identify one relationship that still affects your eating today, what would it be? Why? Think about what it would take to develop closure on that aspect of the relationship. Meditate on being free from the hold that relationship has over your eating.

WEEK 10   🦋   DAY 2

Today's Thin Thought: Food can't fill an empty relationship.

Your daily assignments:
- Drink lots of water.
- Bend, stretch, and use your weights upon waking.
- Walk for at least forty minutes today.
- Keep track of what you put in your mouth.
- Watch your servings/portions.

- Watch your intake of unhealthy fats.
- Move more during the day.
- Choose a variety of whole foods over fragmented foods.
- Take a good multivitamin/multimineral.
- Enhance your diet with nutritional supplements.
- Intentionally pursue a good night's sleep.
- Strategically combat your cravings.
- Cut down on processed sugars.
- **Turn to people, not food.** Relationships should be your source of comfort, excitement, contentment, and satisfaction.

SETTING THE DAY FOR SUCCESS

Yesterday we looked at past relationships. Today I want you to think about the relationships you have right now. These can be with family, friends, coworkers, neighbors. Think about the people around you during the day, the week. How would you characterize these relationships? Are they generally positive? Do you anticipate and enjoy being with these people? Do you participate together in activities and meaningful events? Do you feel connected to others? Do you feel left out and lonely? Do you feel built up and supported by your relationships? Or do you feel drained by them?

Food is a way to fill the void when we don't perceive our present relationships as fulfilling. As we work toward removing food as a way to cope, it makes sense to look at our current relationships and why we think they aren't as supportive as we would like. It may be the relationship has changed over the years, or we entered into it *thinking* it would change but it hasn't. As those relationships changed, food may have rushed in to take its place.

Over the years, your relationship with food may have become your primary relationship. What you eat, how you eat, and how food makes you feel may now constitute a good portion of your daily thought, the way someone who's infatuated romanticizes a lover. Pain when apart, anxiously anticipating the next meeting, remembering the joy of being together—these are ways I have heard people describe their relationship with food. Eating high-fat, high-calorie foods, especially, produce a sensual, almost erotic, pleasure. Remember, this isn't surprising as these foods stimulate the pleasure center of the brain.

It's time to put food back into its proper context of nutrition and reinstate people, real people, as a way to get your relationship needs met.

SUCCESS IN ACTION

I want you to think of all your current relationships. Family, friends, coworkers. Write down the people with whom you're in regular contact. Also write down significant relationships you have, even though you may not actually see that person as much as you'd like. Also make sure to write down "Food" as a relationship. Write the relationships on the left side of your journal. Add three more columns: in the next two, write "Positive" and "Negative." After each identified relationship, indicate what you perceive as good and bad about it. This could be anything from thinking you're not together enough to how that person makes you feel when you are together.

Now it's time for that last column. I want you to head it: "Improvements." Take a look at each of your relationships, including with food, and come up with at least one positive, practical step you can take to improve that relationship. (Be aware there may be a relationship in your mix whose only improvement would be to end it. If that relationship is so negative it outweighs the positives, you may want to seriously consider restricting it or discontinuing it altogether.)

Really take time with this exercise and allow yourself to consider the relationships in your life and how to make them better. When you are proactive, you feel more in charge, more optimistic. The more optimistic and fulfilled you feel in your relationships, the less the siren song of food will entice you to crash your *Thin over 40* goals on the shoals of comfort eating.

WEEK 10 🦋 DAY 3

Today's Thin Thought: Stuffing the pain doesn't make it go away.

Your daily assignments:
- Drink lots of water.
- Bend, stretch, and use your weights upon waking.
- Walk for at least forty minutes today.
- Keep track of what you put in your mouth.
- Watch your servings/portions.
- Watch your intake of unhealthy fats.
- Move more during the day.
- Choose a variety of whole foods over fragmented foods.
- Take a good multivitamin/multimineral.
- Enhance your diet with nutritional supplements.
- Intentionally pursue a good night's sleep.
- Strategically combat your cravings.
- Cut down on processed sugars.
- Turn to people, not food.

Your weekly assignment:
  • Weigh yourself.

SETTING THE DAY FOR SUCCESS

Painful relationships are usually the ones that give us the most trouble, especially when compared to the sure, gratifying result of eating our favorite foods. Whether we're at fault or the other person is, it hurts. So what do you do when someone hurts you? If the usual answer is eat something (rarely broccoli or carrots), it's time to use your maturity and wisdom to devise a different response. Look over the following steps you can take when someone hurts you. (These come from my book *Healing the Scars of Emotional Abuse*. For more information on this book, please see the Resource List in the back.)

• Recognize the offense for what it is. Is it a misunderstanding? Is it intentional? Could it be unintentional? If you're not sure, put your judgment on hold and observe how that person continues to treat you. You may have caught them on a bad day, at a difficult moment.
• Resist the tendency to defend your position. If you determine that you need to confront the other person, offer only your perspective about the incident.
• Give up the need to be right. Allow the other person to concede or to present their own point of view.
• Recognize and apologize for anything you may have done to contribute to the situation. Disagreements are most often a two-way street. A careless remark or misunderstanding on your part might have contributed to the current situation.
• Respond versus react. Learn to be proactive. Stop and evaluate the situation. Reacting immediately,

especially if the other person is not in a responsive mood, can lead to an escalation of tension.

- Seek to build bridges as opposed to either attacking or retreating. A conciliatory attitude is much easier for everyone to deal with than a hostile, defensive one. Practice maintaining an attitude of patience and acceptance. This doesn't mean you agree with what's been done, but rather you choose to respond in a predetermined way.

- Realize you may be the target of someone's anger but not the source of that anger. It simply may not be about you at all. Refuse to take it personally and, thus, magnify the hurt.

- Create your personal limits. You have the right to define what your limits are and to insist that they be respected. Other people may have different limits and will not immediately recognize yours. Explain your limits from the perspective of "I," not "you." In other words, you might begin, "I feel uncomfortable when you speak to me that way . . ." as opposed to "Don't you ever talk to me that way . . ." You have a right to let your objections be heard. It needn't be in an angry, vengeful way, but rather in an assertive, positive way that says, "I respect who I am as a person and I would like you to do the same."

- Remember that even if someone has hurt you, it need not take away your personal happiness (or cause you to seek happiness through food to compensate). You are in charge of your attitude and response. You can get over it and go on (without turning to food).

SUCCESS IN ACTION

As you read over the previous steps, did you identify any that really sound impossible? Any you found yourself trying to argue against? Why do you suppose that is? What did you think would happen if you used these steps in the future? Think back over some major disagreements in your life and relive them, according to those nine steps. The outcome may not have been different, but would you have felt better about yourself if you'd used these steps? You cannot control the reactions of others; you can control your own response.

Take some time today and come up with three alternative responses you're going to use in the future in unpleasant situations with other people. Food cannot be one of them. You might choose instead to calmly reiterate the boundary that person crossed. You might choose to withdraw from the relationship for a short period of time to allow the other person to alter their demeanor. You might choose to go on a walk or engage in another physical activity to work off your sense of frustration with that person.

When dealing with people, hurts and misunderstandings cannot be avoided altogether. It's unrealistic to think they can. By using these steps, you can mitigate their impact and intentionally choose a different response than eating for comfort.

WEEK 10   🦋   DAY 4

Today's Thin Thought: Sometimes it's harder to start from scratch.

Your daily assignments:
- **Drink lots of water.**
- **Bend, stretch, and use your weights upon waking.**
- **Walk for at least forty minutes today.**
- **Keep track of what you put in your mouth.**
- **Watch your servings/portions.**

- Watch your intake of unhealthy fats.
- Move more during the day.
- Choose a variety of whole foods over fragmented foods.
- Take a good multivitamin/multimineral.
- Enhance your diet with nutritional supplements.
- Intentionally pursue a good night's sleep.
- Strategically combat your cravings.
- Cut down on processed sugars.
- Turn to people, not food.

SETTING THE DAY FOR SUCCESS

As you've been thinking about your current relationships, don't fall into the trap of concentrating on the negative. Sure, people are a package deal, but there's also a lot of good that comes in those packages. There's no time like the present, even if you are over forty, to do everything you can to build up and strengthen your current relationships. Over the years, as we get stressed or tired or rushed in daily life, we can take our existing relationships for granted. We think that surely this or that person will understand if we're too tired to communicate or too stressed to participate or too rushed to facilitate. There are times that person will not understand, nor should they. If our relationships are not all we want them to be, we need to take responsibility for our part.

Bad relationships can be a hole where we shovel in food. But it's not just a matter of stopping the food, we also need to see whether or not our actions or lack of action continue to make that hole bigger and bigger. If we don't address the hole itself, the desire to start shoveling food again can trip us up.

It's time to commit to improving our current relationships. We're going to look at six ways to improve relationships today, and six ways tomorrow. You'll be asked to evaluate your current relationships and determine how each of these can make them better.

1. Approach others with an attitude of gentleness and openness. Hostility closes down communication. Think about how you respond to the other person. Do you harbor latent resentment, bitterness, or disappointment toward that person that leaks out in every interaction?

2. When working on a mutual problem, don't assume your solution is the only solution. Respect the other person's point of view and that it could prove invaluable in solving the problem. Again, it's not about you being right; it's about coming to a mutual agreement about the solution.

3. Don't be afraid to speak the truth. Speak it confidently but without a desire to harm the other person. Suppressing a truth can create emotional distress that could trigger a reach for food.

4. Work on being able to separate how you feel about what you say from the message itself. In other words, don't let your emotions overshadow the message. If the message is important enough to convey, take the steps necessary to present it in a way that has the highest chance of being received positively.

5. Be aware of the different ways men and women process information. Men and women often have different worldviews—they may notice different details, or have differing priorities. Accept that a person of the opposite gender may interpret what you say or do differently than it was intended by you. Seek to communicate clearly and openly.

6. Allow the other person to hold an opinion dif-

ferent from yours. Often, we interpret a different opinion as an indictment of our own. This is not always the case. People are allowed to have differing opinions.

SUCCESS IN ACTION

It may seem as if you are the one being asked to do all of the work in strengthening your relationships. You're correct! I want you to realize that it is up to you to do everything you can to build up your relationships. Hopefully, the other person will respond positively and then you'll have their energy added to yours. And it will take your energy, your optimism, your motivation to work on the relationship. During each day, your goal is to look forward to the people around you more than to food.

Look again at the six steps. I want you to choose the one you are best at, and recommit to maintaining that as a positive in your life. Also, choose one that you really need to work on. Evaluate why it is difficult for you to respond that way in a relationship. What are you apprehensive about? Is there a pattern from past relationships that needs to be addressed? Decide how you will respond differently when that situation arises in the future. As your current relationships are strengthened, your need for comfort eating should diminish.

WEEK 10   🦋   DAY 5

Today's Thin Thought: Be accountable for what you say you will do.

Your daily assignments:
- **Drink lots of water.**
- **Bend, stretch, and use your weights upon waking.**

- Walk for at least forty minutes today.
- Keep track of what you put in your mouth.
- Watch your servings/portions.
- Watch your intake of unhealthy fats.
- Move more during the day.
- Choose a variety of whole foods over fragmented foods.
- Take a good multivitamin/multimineral.
- Enhance your diet with nutritional supplements.
- Intentionally pursue a good night's sleep.
- Strategically combat your cravings.
- Cut down on processed sugars.
- Turn to people, not food.

SETTING THE DAY FOR SUCCESS

Today let's continue looking at ways you can strengthen your existing relationships. These should be the main source of comfort and gratification in your life, not food. Food is nourishment and nutrition; it's not the answer for emotional pain. By evaluating and strengthening your relationships, the goal is to reduce the emotional pain you're feeling, as you commit to returning food to its proper context in your life. Let's look over another six ways you can be proactive in maintaining healthy relationships:

1. Always attempt to communicate with an attitude of acceptance—and with love and affection, where applicable. When this is your attitude verbally, it translates into body language, which the other person will read. This attitude opens doors for communication and makes it safe to be open. Think "mercy, grace, and forgiveness" as opposed to "hostility, anger, and frustration."

2. Make sure your motivation to engage in the

conversation is one of enhancing and improving the relationship. Most people don't respond well to mean-spirited criticism. If you do feel you need to bring up a critique, be strategic in how you present it, and when. Bringing it up when the other person feels down or irritable is a surefire opening for an argument, not a discussion. The goal of bringing it up is to provide closure, not blow open the floodgates of a dispute.

3. Allow the other person to make his or her own decisions. This can be especially difficult if you've set in your mind what you're sure they are supposed to do. (This applies to adult relationships. Children are certainly entitled to their own opinion about the situation and should feel free to express them appropriately, but as the parent, or adult, your decision may still need to stand.) You are free to explain your reasons why a certain decision would be the most advantageous, but the other person has the right to decide differently.

4. Seek to inspire trust by extending understanding to the other person and by responding honestly to what is said. It does not build trust in a relationship if you do not express how you truly feel. The other person will eventually pick up on your duplicity and this can strain even the closest relationship.

5. Always be sure to seek forgiveness yourself when you make a mistake. Notice, I didn't say *if* you make a mistake, but *when*. You will make mistakes; everyone does. Don't just pretend it didn't happen and say nothing. Relationships are often built up best through mutual forgiveness. Admitting your own failures will create an atmosphere of openness so other people will feel safer admitting their own mistakes.

6. Be accountable for what you say you will do.

(This is our Thin Thought for the day!) Guilt is one of the strongest negative emotions that can eat away at your insides, provoking a reach for food to numb the pain. Don't feel guilty about not doing what you said you would—just do it, and feel good about yourself!

SUCCESS IN ACTION

Look over these six ways to build up and improve your existing relationships. Identify the one you've got down pat. Identify, also, the one that gives you the most trouble and think about why you have difficulty in this area. Be honest about the roots of this behavior and commit to intentionally responding in a different way.

As a way to help you remember all twelve of these steps, in your journal today look over each of them from yesterday and today and put them into your own short sentence. Over the rest of this week, look them over daily and say them over to yourself. Keep them in mind as you interact with the important people in your life. Work hard to be aware of every interaction you have. Make it positive! And if it isn't, make sure you did all you could to keep it from going sour. If it does, you'll know it wasn't because of anything you did. Then you can let it go and move on.

WEEK 10   🦋   DAY 6

Today's Thin Thought: Sometimes the most beneficial relationship is one that just ended.

Your daily assignments:
- **Drink lots of water.**
- **Bend, stretch, and use your weights upon waking.**

- Walk for at least forty minutes.
- Keep track of what you put in your mouth.
- Watch your servings/portions.
- Watch your intake of unhealthy fats.
- Move more during the day.
- Choose a variety of whole foods over fragmented foods.
- Take a good multivitamin/multimineral.
- Enhance your diet with nutritional supplements.
- Intentionally pursue a good night's sleep.
- Strategically combat your cravings.
- Cut down on processed sugars.
- Turn to people, not food.

SETTING THE DAY FOR SUCCESS

Today, I'd like you to consider any relationship that has such a negative effect on your life it needs to be significantly altered. One of the effects of middle age and beyond can be an honest evaluation of the truths in our lives. This can be difficult, painful, yet necessary. As you've examined past and present relationships this week, I want you to be honest about any that are so negative, so damaging to you as a person, that you need to make changes. The first goal, obviously, is to do what you can to try to move the relationship from mostly negative into a more positive range. This is especially important with core family relationships, which we should do everything possible to hold on to unless they are truly damaging. Unfortunately, there are some people who are toxic, and even being around them becomes so draining you must withdraw from the relationship in order to maintain your own sense of self. Fortunately, most of our relationships, even the negative ones, don't fall into that category.

As you continue to examine your relationships, be aware of any that are extremely negative. Were they always that way, or has the relationship deteriorated over time? Are you able to identify the point at which the relationship soured? Are there specific things you can do to reestablish some of the conditions that made it successful in the first place? For example, what about your relationship with your spouse, your parents, or your children? These are pivotal relationships that reach down to the core of who we are and how we think about ourselves. Restoring these relationships, whenever possible, can be vital to our overall mental health. Especially if these relationships used to be better in the past, it would behoove you to uncover what has changed and what may now be missing in the relationship, and work to restore what's been lost.

It can be easier to make significant changes if the negative relationship is with a coworker, employer, acquaintance, or friend. Leaving a job or a friendship can be easier, in some ways, than ending a familial relationship. Try as you're able to mend the relationship, but if it continues to be a drain on you physically and/or emotionally, consider taking a break from the relationship. If your absence causes the other person to reevaluate their own behavior and decide to make needed changes, your relationship will improve and so will the other person. While it can seem scary to be without that relationship, you may realize there is freedom from the burden it has become.

SUCCESS IN ACTION

As hard as it can be to think about ending a relationship or a friendship, sometimes it's necessary. If you've read this far and realize you don't feel a need to end any relationship you have, take joy in that discovery! And use it recommit yourself to making the most of your relationships. Good relationships are valuable and not to be squandered through neglect or apathy. Be proactive in your relationships. Spend time on them. When you're tempted at night to reach for a piece of cake, reach for the phone instead and call up someone you love. Ask them to help you be accountable for working toward your *Thin over 40* goals. Express gratitude for your relationships and don't shortchange them by seeking the comfort of food instead.

WEEK 10 ❦ DAY 7

Today's Thin Thought: Maybe it's time for a new relationship.

Your daily assignments:
- Drink lots of water.
- Bend, stretch, and use your weights upon waking.
- Walk for at least forty minutes today.
- Keep track of what you put in your mouth.
- Watch your servings/portions.
- Watch your intake of unhealthy fats.
- Move more during the day.
- Choose a variety of whole foods over fragmented foods.
- Take a good multivitamin/multimineral.
- Enhance your diet with nutritional supplements.
- Intentionally pursue a good night's sleep.
- Strategically combat your cravings.
- Cut down on processed sugars.
- Turn to people, not food.

Weekly Assignment:
  • Go grocery shopping for next week.

SETTING THE DAY FOR SUCCESS

After looking over your current relationships, you may realize you don't have as many significant ones as you'd like. Or perhaps your relationships are focused on the negative and you see the need for more positive relationships in your life. While it is possible to turn negative relationships into positive, there is another way to bring those positives in. Consider seeking out and creating a new relationship. This will be especially true if you've had some important relationships end, either through death, divorce, a change in location, or a change in job. You may not have realized the void this left in your life, a void you've been filling up with food. Perhaps it's time to get into the world again and establish some new relationships.

SUCCESS IN ACTION

If you are looking for a new relationship in your life, there are many places you can go to meet new people and establish connections. This needn't be a romantic involvement, but you could be looking for someone your own age you can relate to, someone younger to mentor, or an older person from whom you can gain experience. Evaluate your life and your relationships and see if there's a space you'd like to fill up with a new relationship. Think about what that space represents to you. Where is a person like that most likely to be found? Remember, one of the best ways to make a friend is to be one yourself. Look for volunteer opportunities in your civic or faith community. Open yourself up to other people.

Getting out more and involving yourself with others can help you meet new people and detach you from your emotional relationship with food.

HERO OF THE WEEK

My Hero this week is a woman I'll call Patricia. Patricia is in her sixties and has lived a life of loss. She's been divorced for years and her children are grown and live out of state. Over the years, she mourned the loss of the significant relationships in her life. The people who did come into her life didn't stay long because of her immense need to be accepted and cared for. She burned people up, and each fractured new relationship brought back the pain of old ones. So desperate was she to fill up the emotional void, she turned to food as a source of comfort. Patricia lived in a cycle of increasing weight, increasing health problems, and decreasing positive interaction with others.

Patricia is my Hero of the Week because she has taken responsibility for this pattern. Through counseling, she is working through her issues with food and her dependence upon other people. She's working on returning food to its proper place of nutrition. She's learning about the way her body functions and what she can do to help as she ages. Patricia's also taking a good, hard look at the way she's been relating to other people. Making changes isn't easy, but she's committed to doing so. Along the way, she's feeling better physically and about herself, and painful relationships are being mended. She thought she was too old to change. Patricia's learning to love herself again and enjoy life!

WEEK 11
MAKING THE MOST OF FORGIVENESS

WEEK 11 ❧ DAY 1

Today's Thin Thought: Two steps forward and one step back is still progress.

Congratulations on reaching Week 11 in *Thin over 40*! This is a pivotal week because we're going to deal with that inevitable occurrence—the backslide, the "one step back." Because it is inevitable, it's vital that you accept it and plan to successfully navigate around it. One of the most successful strategies for handling a backslide is understanding the proper role of forgiveness. That's why Forgiveness is this week's Key Concept.

Your daily assignments: (Say them aloud to yourself each day. Listen to your voice and agree with yourself how important these are.)

- **Drink lots of water.** We're mostly water and need it for every life function.
- **Bend, stretch, and use your weights upon waking.** Help your body help you accomplish your goals.
- **Walk for at least forty minutes today.** Don't feel guilty about this time for yourself.
- **Keep track of what you put in your mouth.** Be aware of how your choices affect how you feel.

214

- **Watch your servings/portions.** And watch that excess weight come off.
- **Watch your intake of unhealthy fats.** Make smart choices about the types and amounts of fats.
- **Move more during the day.** Keep your body active. Sit up! Be physically alert.
- **Choose a variety of whole foods over fragmented foods.** All those skins and husks are packed with nutrients—don't shortchange yourself.
- **Take a good multivitamin/multimineral.**
- **Enhance your diet with nutritional supplements.** Give your body what it needs and you'll feel better.
- **Intentionally pursue a good night's sleep.** Learn to enjoy the process of falling asleep again.
- **Strategically combat your cravings.** Ask yourself what you *really* need and find a healthy way to provide it.
- **Cut down on processed sugars.** Wean your body from processed sugars.
- **Turn to people, not food.** Continue your good work on sorting out the tie between your relationships to others and your relationship to food.

SETTING THE DAY FOR SUCCESS

While being over forty has tremendous advantages, there can be an age-related disadvantage—desperation. Desperation can produce all-or-nothing thinking. To put it another way, you need to guard against the idea that you've got to get this *Thin over 40* thing down pat immediately because time is running out and if it doesn't happen now it's not going to ever happen because you've tried it a dozen times before and nothing's ever worked long-term and you've just about given up hope but you've put yourself out on a limb to try one last time and if you're unable to pull it together to do it this time, well, just forget it.

Do you see my point? Once you allow yourself to enter the downward spiral of all-or-nothing thinking, your ultimate destination is nothing. This is because, being fallible human beings, we're not able to pull off "all" all the time. Our life is a series of forward and backward steps. Our goal is to make more forward steps than backward. But if we think we can completely eliminate the backward, we're kidding ourselves and setting ourselves up for the failure of unrealistic expectations.

We need to recognize who we really are, not who we think we ought to be. Too many of us have grown up with the idea that we need to be perfect to be acceptable to ourselves and others. We've strived and strained, prodded and pulled ourselves through life attempting to achieve perfection and beating ourselves up when we didn't reach it. This can be especially true in our health goals. We may be successful in so many other areas of life, yet feel a failure because we're over forty and out of shape.

Desperation obscures reality and it also confuses time. We expect to have immediate, dramatic results. When progress takes twice as long as we planned (because of that one-step-back-for-every-two-steps-forward thing), we determine that we're only half as successful as we should be. Instead of seeing two steps forward and one step back as progress, we see it as regression because we expected to be two steps forward and we're only one. Because progress doesn't match our ideal of success, we see it as failure. It becomes, then, a matter of perception. Do we think we've failed? Yes! Have we really failed? No, we've gone forward! We need to base our perception firmly in reality.

SUCCESS IN ACTION

Each day this week in the Success in Action section, you're going to take a realistic look at a backsliding scenario. Even if the scenario presented is not one that totally corresponds to your situation, please work through the strategies for success anyway. There is value to be gained even when everything doesn't completely line up. That's life, remember?

One of the most common backslides begins by starting out the day with good intentions and ending it with broken promises to yourself. It seems like you've got all the willpower in the world when you're at work and distracted, but once you hit that comfort zone called home, all bets are off. Being so "good" during the day can even be used against you. You figure you're allowed to relax a little in the evening. One serving at dinner becomes two or three. In the later evening, out come the chips, the cookies, the ice cream, even if you're not hungry. You determine you'll just have a little bit and, after all, a little bit won't hurt. That half cup of ice cream becomes a full bowl. Two cookies become half a dozen. That handful of chips becomes half a bag.

Before you know it, you're a step back on a twostep day. Now is the time to learn from the situation, not allow it to destroy your resolve. Let's look at what is the perception and the reality of this situation. Think about what your perceptions are as you head into the evening. They probably look something like this: (1) Being good during the day means you

can be just a little bad at night; (2) Home is where
you can relax your commitments to yourself; (3) Even
if you start, you should be able to stop by now. (Go
ahead and add your own, as you think about a personal, similar situation.)

Now, think about the reality. First, *Thin over 40*
isn't about leveraging the "good" against the "bad."
It's about making healthy choices based on nutrition,
not reward. Second, home is a wonderful place to
relax, but your commitments to yourself transcend
location. And third, you need to give yourself more
time to work through your issues with certain foods
or habits before you indulge in them. This isn't deprivation, it's wisdom.

WEEK 11   ❦   DAY 2

*Today's Thin Thought: Giant leaps are great,
but most progress is made by baby steps.*

Your daily assignments:
- Drink lots of water.
- Bend, stretch, and use your weights upon
  waking.
- Walk for at least forty minutes today.
- Keep track of what you put in your mouth.
- Watch your servings/portions.
- Watch your intake of unhealthy fats.
- Move more during the day.
- Choose a variety of whole foods over frag-
  mented foods.
- Take a good multivitamin/multimineral.
- Enhance your diet with nutritional supple-
  ments.
- Intentionally pursue a good night's sleep.
- Strategically combat your cravings.
- Cut down on processed sugars.

- Turn to people, not food.
- Focus on your progress.

SETTING THE DAY FOR SUCCESS

If we're honest with ourselves, most of us want progress in great, leaping strides. We'd really like to be a champion long jumper when it comes to our goals—running full bore, launching ourselves into the air of freedom, and landing yards from where we started! We want to be the hare, not the tortoise. Giant leaps sound so much better than baby steps. We assume, as adults, that we should operate beyond baby steps.

Let's look at it another way. If you have children (if you don't, think of a friend's child or a niece or nephew), what was your reaction when he or she took that first step? Were you incensed that they weren't farther along? Did you critique the form or castigate the wobbliness? (I should certainly hope not!) On the contrary, your first reaction was to cheer! You had a realistic understanding of just what it takes to walk on your own and you were amazed, pleased, and proud when your child accomplished that milestone.

With both my children, I can remember vividly watching those first tentative steps. I couldn't seem to keep quiet; I was so excited and pleased, all I wanted to do was encourage my boys. After all, it's an important, worthwhile skill, and I could tell from their faces they were trying so hard. I didn't expect them to be able to run before they learned to walk. I took each step for what it was—a real high point in their physical and even emotional development. Learning to walk is a physical milestone, but it's also an emotional milestone in that it supports the natural independence of a child that age. Understanding what was at stake, how could I do anything but cheer them on?

Are you treating yourself that way as you work toward each milestone in *Thin over 40*? Are you cheering yourself on? Or are you standing on the mental sidelines shaking your head over your own baby steps? After all, there's a great similarity between your child integrating the new skill of walking and you integrating the new skills of a healthier lifestyle. The similarity is that new skills take time and practice to mature. Instead of disparaging the idea of baby steps, relive those wonderful moments in your own life when you mastered a skill or habit—and cheer yourself on!

SUCCESS IN ACTION

In your journal today, I want you to write yourself a pep talk for those times you doubt your progress. I want you to cheer yourself on by complimenting your growth. Recognize the good things you've learned and done. Give yourself a big star, happy face, or exclamation point, whatever conveys that you're proud of yourself and understand the reality of your progress. Don't look down on yourself for taking baby steps. Your goal isn't to be perfect; it's to get stronger, steadier, and surer of yourself as you gain experience.

WEEK 11   🦋   DAY 3

Today's Thin Thought: If you think you're a failure, you will fail.

Your daily assignments:
  • **Drink lots of water.**

- Bend, stretch, and use your weights upon waking.
- Walk for at least forty minutes today.
- Keep track of what you put in your mouth.
- Watch your servings/portions.
- Watch your intake of unhealthy fats.
- Move more during the day.
- Choose a variety of whole foods over fragmented food.
- Take a good multivitamin/multimineral.
- Enhance your diet with nutritional supplements.
- Intentionally pursue a good night's sleep.
- Strategically combat your cravings.
- Cut down on processed sugars.
- Turn to people, not food.
- Focus on your progress.

Your weekly assignment:
- Weigh yourself.

SETTING THE DAY FOR SUCCESS

Sometimes we feel the biggest failure when we step off those dreaded bathroom scales. If we thought we should have lost at least three pounds and all we see is a pound less, we tell ourselves we've just gained two pounds! Live by the scale, die by the scale, and we seem to do more dying than living.

Wallowing in self-defeat is a major backslide. Feeling defeated drains you of motivation. It calls into question the energy and drive required to maintain forward momentum. If you're already defeated, what's the point of going on? The logical thing to do is admit defeat and try to live with it. Of course, that's the problem—you can't really live with defeat.

Constant defeat makes an unhealthy life partner and is incompatible with the *Thin over 40* lifestyle.

In order to move beyond those inevitable backward steps, you must see yourself as an overall success. It's far too easy for any of us to concentrate on the negative, and your particular upbringing may have supremely prepared you for thinking the worst about yourself. You need to rewrite those internal tapes in your head that play over and over that all this work is useless because you'll never be able to do it anyway.

If you're convinced you're going to fail, you will. That's because you'll actually be working to bring about the expected result. You'll eat things you know you shouldn't because you'll figure, what's the point? Old habits will continue to maintain their stranglehold on you because you figure they're so strong you'll never be able to break free. Any setback along the way you'll regard as proof of the folly of this whole endeavor. You look at the discomfort of dealing with your failure and think it in no way compensates for the loss of comfort that food brings. You conclude you'd rather get comfort from food than none at all.

Can you see where this poisonous line of thinking gets you? When you've predetermined that failure is inevitable, it will be. When people come to my clinic to overcome the bondage of an eating disorder, we ask each of them to do something extremely difficult. We ask them to believe in their ability to get better. Without it, there's little we can do. In my almost twenty years of counseling, I can tell you that if a person comes into the recovery process convinced they cannot, or determined they will not, get better, recovery is extremely rare. If there's even the smallest spark of hope, of belief in a better future, we're able to fan that into the warmth of recovery. If it's not there, we've got very little to work from. But when the seeds of hope exist, even in short supply, an amazing harvest of recovery can occur.

SUCCESS IN ACTION

I want you to be really honest about the barriers to success you erect yourself. You've got to be your own best supporter! Others can assist you, but you've got to believe in your ability to change.

In your journal today, at the top of the page, I want you to draw a flame, entitled "Hope." Underneath that flame, I want you to draw two columns. On top of the left column, draw a piece of wood. On top of the right column, draw a bucket of water. Under the wood, list out all of the positive steps you're taking to keep yourself encouraged and motivated throughout *Thin over 40*. Each baby step adds fuel to the fire! Honestly list under the bucket of water all the ways you're acting as a wet blanket to that hope. How are you defeating your efforts? Your goal this week is to take the fresh wind of optimism and fan your flame of hope!

WEEK 11 🦋 DAY 4

Today's Thin Thought: Life can be managed, not contained.

Your daily assignments:
- **Drink lots of water.**
- **Bend, stretch, and use your weights upon waking.**
- **Walk for at least forty minutes today.**
- **Keep track of what you put in your mouth.**
- **Watch your servings/portions.**
- **Watch your intake of unhealthy fats.**

- Move more during the day.
- Choose a variety of whole foods over fragmented foods.
- Take a good multivitamin/multimineral.
- Enhance your diet with nutritional supplements.
- Intentionally pursue a good night's sleep.
- Strategically combat your cravings.
- Cut down on processed sugars.
- Turn to people, not food.
- Focus on your progress.

SETTING THE DAY FOR SUCCESS

Today let's look at another potent friend of backsliding—self-pity. In other words, you look around you at people who don't seem to have as much of a problem with their weight and health as you do and complain, *Why me*? You blame your job, your family, your kids, your upbringing, your metabolism, your body shape for foisting such a burden on you. It's unfair; it's not right. Since they find it so easy to maintain a healthy weight, why should you be the one who always has to struggle? Their situation doesn't seem to be nearly as hard as yours.

Even if that's true, it's irrelevant where your situation is concerned! Your situation is unique and only you can work within that situation to bring about positive change.

Today we're going to go over the components of the Serenity Prayer, popularized by many self-help groups. It goes like this: "God, grant me the serenity to accept the things I cannot change; courage to change the things I can; and wisdom to know the difference." What this prayer basically says is that life can be managed but not contained. There are always going to be things in life we cannot change but must accept. On the other side, it acknowledges that our condition in life is not immutable, we can affect change. The beauty and desire, of course, is to know the difference.

Now, there are certain aspects you cannot change. For example, if you are a person with a large frame, you will not be able to fit into a size-four dress or a thirty waist. Nor would you want to! There is a healthy size and weight for your body type and that should be your goal, not trying to look like someone else you've decided has the "perfect" body. Wallowing in self-pity because you're not a size four isn't likely to make you a size four; it's more likely to make you a size twenty.

If you started this process seventy pounds beyond a healthy weight for you, it will take a longer period of time for you to lose that weight than someone who wants to lose twenty or thirty pounds. This isn't a race; it isn't a competition; it's not overnight. Losing weight in a healthful manner takes a certain amount of time.

Complicating your desire to change your weight may be the reality of a disability or condition that hinders physical exercise. Simply put, it may be difficult for you to get out and exercise. Your condition may require you to make modifcations to your home or go to a location that is prepared to assist you with exercise. While this adds inconvenience, please do not allow it to dissuade you from your goal of increased physical health. Keep striving toward your goals and refuse to sink into self-pity. Take advantage of community resources through a local hospital, gym, or rehabilitation center. If you cannot drive, ask a friend or acquaintance, or look into the possibility of public transportation. You won't know what you're able to accomplish until you try. You do know you'll accomplish little if you quit.

Let's look at the second component of to this prayer. It can take courage to acknowledge what needs to be changed and actually change. Many of us resist change because of the effort involved, especially if we've convinced ourselves that change will be too difficult. Courage says to go ahead and start the process anyway, even with the understanding that it's not going to be easy. It took a certain amount of courage to pick up this book. It takes even more to read it, and even more to actively participate in it. Starting from where you are, work toward increasing your courage. You do this by accepting the guidelines, suggestions and insights in this book and putting them into practice in your life. You'll gain courage as you see success.

Wisdom is the third component of this prayer. So often, we spin our wheels trying in vain to change the unchangeable. This diverts our attention and energy away from changing those things we really can. We end up no better for all that effort; in fact, we fare worse, assured of the inevitability of our own failure. Failure was inevitable because we set out to change the wrong thing.

SUCCESS IN ACTION

In your journal, I want you to look at your life in light of this Serenity Prayer. Divide a piece of paper into three sections. In one, write down those things about yourself that you cannot change. On the top of this section, write "Acceptance." You can list physical characteristics, family realities, concrete events in your life.

In another, write down those things about yourself that are subject to change. On top of this section, write "Courage," to remind you what it will take to actually implement those changes. On top of the last section, write "Wisdom." In this section you're going to write down all of the things that didn't immediately fall into the other two categories. These are either physical aspects or personality traits that you would like to change but aren't sure about. Over the next several days, I want you to meditate on these aspects and try to come to some conclusion about which of the other categories each should be in. For those that are really puzzling, consider obtaining counsel from a friend or professional. Often, their insight can prove invaluable in helping you answer the difficult questions.

WEEK 11 🦋 DAY 5

Today's Thin Thought: Forgiveness isn't a free pass.

Your daily assignments:
- Drink lots of water.
- Bend, stretch, and use your weights upon waking.
- Walk for at least forty minutes today.
- Keep track of what you put in your mouth.
- Watch your servings/portions.
- Watch your intake of unhealthy fats.
- Move more during the day.
- Choose a variety of whole foods over fragmented foods.
- Take a good multivitamin/multimineral.
- Enhance your diet with nutritional supplements.
- Intentionally pursue a good night's sleep.
- Strategically combat your cravings.
- Cut down on processed sugars.

- Turn to people, not food.
- Focus on your progress.

SETTING THE DAY FOR SUCCESS

This week we've been looking at significant road-blocks, or backslides, along the way to a *Thin over 40* life. And we've been talking quite a bit about the concept of forgiveness and how beneficial it can be. There is a sinkhole, however, along this road that has forgiveness written all over it. Of course, it might say "forgiveness," but it's been mislabeled. Instead, it should read "denial." Here's what happens: You backslide a little and "forgive" yourself, only to find that you have to continually "forgive" yourself for the very same thing, over and over again. You can't understand why this aspect of your life isn't getting any better. You're forgiving yourself and you're expecting to move on—but you're stuck.

I believe the key lies in understanding the mechanism of forgiveness. In order to forgive yourself, there needs to be an acceptance that what you've done should be changed. To use a religious word, in order for forgiveness to take place, there must first be repentance. It's a little hard to accept forgiveness from someone if you don't really think you've done anything wrong in the first place! It's no different with you. If, deep down, you don't acknowledge what you've been doing is detrimental, there's no real repentance and forgiveness becomes moot.

Now, why wouldn't you accept that something obviously not good for you is really detrimental? Because you've ascribed that behavior with so many positives they outweigh the obvious negatives. In other words, if you have decided that it is beneficial for you to start your day off with a high-calorie, high-caffeine drink because you just can't get going any other way, you're more likely to overlook the hypoglycemic crash that occurs midmorning. Or, if you've come to the conclusion that it's beneficial to be able to stop at a fast-food outlet for lunch each day because of your hectic schedule, you'll tend to overlook the fact that your cholesterol counts keep coming in high.

This can also occur in the opposite. In other words, you can ascribe to a positive behavior so many negatives, it actually becomes a negative in your mind. Exercise is a prime example of this. If you have decided that it's too much of a bother, too inconvenient, or too unrealistic for you to get out and exercise each day, you won't. Even though exercise is essential and beneficial, you'll keep seeing it through your negative lenses and it simply won't happen consistently. Refusing to see positive things as positive and negative things as negative is called "denial." When forgiveness acts like a free pass allowing you to continue detrimental behavior, it's not forgiveness, it's denial. The antidote for denial is truth.

SUCCESS IN ACTION

Think about your entrenched backslides or places where you're finding it especially difficult to adhere to what you've learned in *Thin over 40*. Examine how you really feel about those activities. Is it just a case of forgiving yourself and moving on? Or, are you really just hanging on to those behaviors because you still see them as a benefit to you?

Write down two or three areas you need to honestly evaluate. Do you really want to give up those behaviors? Why do you think you're having such a struggle working past them? Are you willing to do what it takes to bring about change where these areas are concerned? If so, explain your motivation for change. If not, be honest about what benefit those behaviors give you. Are there other ways to meet those needs, without engaging in those behaviors? What is holding you back? What do you need to focus on, in order to find the courage to change?

WEEK 11 🦋 DAY 6

Today's Thin Thought: Forgiveness forges a pathway around guilt.

Your daily assignments:
- Drink lots of water.
- Bend, stretch, and use your weights upon waking.
- Walk for at least forty minutes today.
- Keep track of what you put in your mouth.
- Watch your servings/portions.
- Watch your intake of unhealthy fats.
- Move more during the day.
- Choose a variety of whole foods over fragmented foods.
- Take a good multivitamin/multimineral.
- Enhance your diet with nutritional supplements.
- Intentionally pursue a good night's sleep.
- Strategically combat your cravings.
- Cut down on processed sugars.
- Turn to people, not food.
- Focus on your progress.

SETTING THE DAY FOR SUCCESS

There are perhaps no greater weights on progress than guilt and shame. These twin voices scream their support of self-pity and call out against forgiveness.

Guilt and shame combine to produce intense feelings of anger—at the situation, at other people, and at you. Working through these powerful emotions can be a key to success. When you experience guilt, you're focusing on your perceived failures and it's difficult to see your way clear to view success. You may feel guilty about how you've "let yourself go." You may feel guilty about your relationship with food. You may feel guilt over the amount of time, energy, and money you've invested over the years in controlling your weight. That guilt may very well have argued against buying or working through this book. Every unsuccessful attempt to deal with the guilt becomes a source of shame.

Shame is an incredibly powerful emotion that can cause absolute paralysis where positive change is concerned. Shame insists that you're not worth the effort and that any present or future negatives are compensation for past shame. You may be ashamed of the way you look. Ashamed of the way you eat. Ashamed of your own "weakness" for allowing yourself to wind up in your present condition. If you're experiencing physical concerns due to your health, you may be ashamed of the resources being used to address them. Whatever the source of your shame, it's acting as an anchor around your progress, pulling you down. You need to forgive yourself, cut the rope, and move forward.

So how do you know if your feelings of guilt and shame require true forgiveness, or if you're caught in the false trap of denial? When guilt and shame are present, there is no question as to feelings of remorse. There's no question that deep down you feel as if you've done wrong. In fact, you are so overcome with remorse, you feel repentance is useless because forgiveness is impossible. You've messed things up so badly, you're in no position to expect forgiveness from others or extend forgiveness to yourself. This attitude keeps you stuck in the very behaviors you want to change. It provides you no way out.

The only way to get beyond guilt and shame is to risk the act of self-forgiveness and rekindle a positive view of self. When you do this, you dissipate much of the unresolved anger you feel. Over time, guilt and shame become such a burden, the mind backlashes against them, often through misdirected anger. This anger can fuel a misconception that positive change is a useless gesture. This anger can find itself redirected toward close associates and family. It can also fuel the feeling of rebellion that says trying to control your weight is oppressive in nature and you should be able to eat what and how much you want. Dealing with any residual anger, guilt, and shame is vital to continued progress in your *Thin over 40* goals.

SUCCESS IN ACTION

Often guilt and shame lie hidden in the background of your mind so it can be difficult to identify them. Today I want you to answer the following questions, once with your first initial response and again after some time for personal reflection:

- As I look back over my life, I still feel guilty about . . .
- Viewing my life today, I am most ashamed about . . .
- When I think about who I am right now, it makes me angry to think that I still . . .

Write down both responses and really evaluate your answers and how these feelings interfere with your optimism, motivation, and commitment to live a healthier life.

WEEK 11 🦋 DAY 7

Today's Thin Thought: Forgiveness allows you to focus on the future.

Your daily assignments:
- Drink lots of water.
- Bend, stretch, and use your weights upon waking.
- Walk for at least forty minutes today.
- Keep track of what you put in your mouth.
- Watch your servings/portions.
- Watch your intake of unhealthy fats.
- Move more during the day.
- Choose a variety of whole foods over fragmented foods.
- Take a good multivitamin/multimineral.
- Enhance your diet with nutritional supplements.
- Intentionally pursue a good night's sleep.
- Strategically combat your cravings.
- Cut down on processed sugars.
- Turn to people, not food.
- Focus on your progress.

Weekly Assignment:
- Go grocery shopping for next week.

SETTING THE DAY FOR SUCCESS

When we keep our minds centered on the backward steps in our past and present, we neglect to focus on the promise the forward steps hold for the future—because we are moving forward. And if we'll just keep at it, we're going to end up where we want to be! Granted, we may not get there as quickly as we thought or as easily as we wanted but, in the final analysis, will either of those be an issue when we're celebrating our goals? No! Instead we'll be enjoying our victories after learning from our struggles.

Keep focused on those forward steps, while learning from the backward ones. Your goal is to minimize the times those backward steps trip you up. And when it does happen, for it will, view each misstep for what it truly is, be honest with yourself always, forgive yourself when necessary, and move on! Commit to integrating more of the *Thin over 40* lifestyle each day. Allow yourself to take those baby steps necessary to see the progress you desire. Don't burden yourself with unrealistic expectations, denial, anger, guilt, or shame. When you recognize the weight of one of these holding you back, work to detach it and keep going.

Be aware that you may find you are having difficulty working through some of these negative emotions. Difficult does not mean impossible, but I want you to be open to the possibility that speaking with a counselor or therapist might prove to be just the support you need to work through some entrenched feelings holding you back. Now, please withstand any temptations you might feel to view counseling with shame or guilt! There is no shame in going to a therapist, and I don't say this merely because that is my profession. It has been in therapy sessions where I have seen the most stunning examples of courage and perseverance ever. I feel privileged to assist people in finding their own core of courage and the strength to move beyond very difficult circumstances and emotions. My role as a therapist is not to "cure" people but to help each person find the strength within themselves—that I know is there—to move toward a better life and a better future.

SUCCESS IN ACTION

Imagine yourself going to speak to a counselor or therapist. Do you perceive this as a positive experience? If so, why? What would you like to work on? If not, can you identify where those negative impressions come from? Do you consider counseling to be an admission of weakness? If not a counselor, would you consider speaking to a trusted mentor or friend?

Write down the name of someone you feel you could confide in and trust to assist you in working through tough feelings of denial, anger, guilt, or shame. You may not have the need or feel ready right now to take advantage of that name, but I'd like you to go ahead and write it down in case circumstances change in the future. All of us should be able to identify a safe person we can share difficult issues with.

HERO OF THE WEEK

Imagine a thin version of yourself visible for everyone to see, right next to you. As if you're always the "before" and the "after" follows you around wherever you go, reminding other people how far it is between the two. This was Jan's experience growing up as a twin. Jan's twin was always a thin version of herself. All through school, in every picture, in every situation, other people were able to see what Jan would look like if only she were thinner. Being twins, Jan and her sister did look very much alike, but Jan became known as "the fat one."

To her credit, Jan's twin never concentrated on Jan's weight or made it an issue between them. But Jan did, even if she didn't always articulate it. As an adult, Jan would feel such shame because she weighed more than her twin. She never seemed to be able to be as thin and Jan saw this as a major weakness in her life, feeling guilty and allowing this as a wedge in her relationship with her sister.

I remember asking her to bring in pictures of them both growing up. After a bit of digging, she brought in several and we spread them out on a table. You see, Jan was operating under the assumption that she was supposed to be an *identical* twin. From the pictures, it was obvious that Jan and her sister were *fraternal*, a fact she readily admitted. Even though Jan knew they were really fraternal, she assumed they were supposed to look identical because they looked similar. Jan, even from childhood, obviously had a different face and body shape. Her twin was always thinner, even when they were babies.

It came as a revelation to Jan that all these years she'd developed guilt and shame over her body, based upon a misconception. Jan's my Hero of the Week because she found the courage to let go of that perception and learn to accept herself for who she truly is. It has given her the courage to let go of the anger and the comfort behavior she'd developed with food to deal with that anger. Her relationship with herself is blossoming and her relationship with her sister has never been better.

WEEK 12
MAKING THE MOST OF LIFE

WEEK 12   🦋   DAY 1

Today's Thin Thought: In for a penny, in for a pound.

Today marks the beginning of your twelfth week training for your *Thin over 40* life. This week, I want you to focus on that word—"beginning." Even in your twelfth week, you're still beginning to integrate the principles and apply them to your individual situation, to your life. What you are learning is for the long haul and will continue to have health-enhancing, life-changing results from this week forward.

During this week, our Key Concept is Success. Focus on the success you've enjoyed over the past eleven weeks and commit yourself to continued success as you live each day *Thin over 40*. We're also going to look at those challenge areas and help you strategize around them.

Your daily assignments: *(These are your components for success. Don't shortchange them, but take them fully to heart! This week, I've shortened them to help you memorize them.)*
- **Drink lots of water.**
- **Use your body upon waking.**
- **Walk for forty-five minutes.**

- Keep track of what and how much you eat.
- Choose healthy fats in moderation.
- Be physically active during the day.
- Choose whole foods.
- Take a multivitamin.
- Take nutritional supplements.
- Get a good night's sleep.
- Combat your cravings.
- Cut down on sugar.
- Turn to people, not food.
- Focus on your success.

SETTING THE DAY FOR SUCCESS

Every day during this training, we've talked about success. We've thought about what success means to you. Today I'd like you to think about it again. I'd like you to focus on it and anchor yourself in it. Many times, people begin to make dietary and lifestyle changes, thinking that they can put up with "anything" for a short amount of time. Already, they perceive their efforts as going toward something negative, something they must endure. If there is anything I'd like you to get out of this twelve-week training it's that these changes are not negative!

I cannot tell you the number of newspaper and magazine articles I've read about our increasingly overweight population. As a country, we are getting fatter. There's an idea that all people need is information and that will cause the country to see the light of good nutrition. Now, I believe in the value of good information and have worked to include the very latest within each week. (Please see the Resource List at the back of this book, for a variety of further materials for you to take advantage of.

There is nutritional information everywhere, from

food packaging to headlines, about the latest discovery. It seems like every morning when we wake up, someone else wants to tell us what to eat, what not to eat, when to eat, how to eat. Yet with all of the emphasis on nutrition and food, we still get larger and larger as a country. No, I don't think information alone is the key to success. Rather, I believe that understanding is the true key. Over the last eleven weeks, you've been increasing your understanding of the following:

- Food and its various components
- How your body works, especially over age forty
- How your emotions and faulty beliefs are tied to food
- How your upbringing established eating patterns
- How food has intersected your stress coping mechanisms
- What success means to you

When you understand yourself, your situation, your eating patterns, your body, you are able to take all of this information and filter it into components that make sense for you. It needn't be that complicated. We *make* it complicated, often because we really don't want to take the steps necessary to bring about positive change in our lives. We'd rather search for exceptions and strategize loopholes in order to still do what we want. For the vast majority of us, the reason we're overweight is because we eat too much of some foods, too little of others, and don't use our bodies enough. As a result, we are overweight and feel lousy, emotionally and physically. The joy of *Thin over 40* is that you don't have to continue in that pattern. You've been taking positive steps to come out of that unhealthy lifestyle and proactively pursue a different course for yourself for middle age and beyond. Keep with that commitment!

SUCCESS IN ACTION

Using short phrases and statements, look at the six topics you've been learning. Personalize them. Under each, write down what comes to the forefront of your mind. For example, under "Emotions and faulty beliefs," you might write, "When I feel marginalized at home or work, I turn to sweets." Or, under "Eating patterns growing up," you might write, "I've learned I eat a lot of food in a hurry now because growing up in a large family, there was rarely enough food to go around."

This is a time for reflection and putting on paper the various insights you've gained over the past eleven weeks. Today, do this literally off the top of your head. It isn't some sort of a test where you're supposed to subcategorize everything. Those thoughts that have made the greatest impact are the ones that will probably come to mind first. These are the ones you don't need to review because you carry them around on the surface of your mind already.

WEEK 12   🦋   DAY 2

Today's Thin Thought: Learn to get more bang for your caloric buck.

Your daily assignments: *(Work on memorizing these thirteen short statements in order to be able to recall them at will when you need to remind yourself of the components of the* Thin over 40 *plan. In fact, let's personalize them.)*

- I drink lots of water.
- I use my body upon waking.
- I walk for at least forty-five minutes a day.

- I keep track of what I eat and how much.
- I choose healthy fats in moderation.
- I am physically active.
- I eat whole foods.
- I take my vitamins.
- I take my supplements.
- I get a good night's sleep.
- I combat my cravings.
- I cut down on sugar.
- I turn to people, not food.
- I focus on my success.

SETTING THE DAY FOR SUCCESS

Today I'd like you to recommit yourself to feeding your body only, to really look at the food you eat as the fuel burned for energy and used for repair and maintenance of a truly remarkable physical system. It doesn't matter how old you are or with what conditions, your body is still fascinating, complex, and remarkable! And what you put into it really does matter. Up to now, you may have discovered that your emotions, or advertising, or habits, or convenience determined what you put into your body. Your continued assignment is to let your *body* and its needs be in charge of what you eat. Your emotions aren't concerned with your physicality. Advertisers could care less about what's good for you; they're in it for what's good for them. Habits are done on autopilot and, over forty, somebody's got to be at the helm! Convenience is only interested in the here and now, not the consequences down the road.

We've bought into the lie that it has to be fast, sweet, salty, or fatty to taste good. We've been conditioned into believing the best things in life come out of a plastic wrapper. Your goal for *Thin over 40* is to continue to prove those misconceptions wrong. Eat well by eating healthy. Give your body what it needs and allow it to reward you with renewed energy, stabilized moods, increased stamina, and a zest for life!

SUCCESS IN ACTION

In your journal today, I want you to tell your old way of thinking about food and eating good-bye. Understand that how you view and deal with food is a *relationship*. You're leaving your old relationship with food behind and committing to your new one. You've had almost three months to get to know this new relationship and it's time to fully commit to it, if you have not already. Be bold and honest, however, about the truth of what you'll miss and what you won't about your old relationship with food. Thank food for helping you through whatever difficulties it did in the past, but acknowledge that those positives have been far outweighed by the negatives you now find in your life. Let your old relationship know you're ready to move on. Praise your new relationship with food and all of its advantages. Purposefully put the past behind you and commit to the future—your healthy *Thin over 40* future!

WEEK 12   🦋   DAY 3

*Today's Thin Thought: Accepting your age
helps you age gracefully.*

Your daily assignments:
- I drink lots of water.
- I use my body upon waking.
- I walk for at least forty-five minutes a day.
- I keep track of what I eat and how much.
- I choose healthy fats in moderation.

- I am physically active.
- I eat whole foods.
- I take my vitamins.
- I take my supplements.
- I get a good night's sleep.
- I combat my cravings.
- I cut down on sugar.
- I turn to people, not food.
- I focus on my success.

Your weekly assignment:
- Weigh yourself.

SETTING THE DAY FOR SUCCESS

How do you age gracefully? Does that indicate some sort of defeat? How do you feel about "growing old?" Frightened? Frustrated? Apprehensive? Angry? These are important questions because they point to your attitude about your over-forty body.

I'd also like you to think about another important question—how do you feel about death? Many people are stuck in denial about their physical bodies over forty because they don't want to acknowledge the aging process. They don't want to acknowledge the aging process because they equate aging with death. They don't want to die, therefore, they don't want to age. Denial of aging becomes a way of denying the reality of death. Perversely, their denial of aging and failure to take aging into account in their lifestyles hastens the very thing they're afraid of. Obesity and lack of exercise lead to premature death through heart disease, stroke, and diabetes.

Thin over 40 cannot make you live forever, but it can help you sustain vibrant health into your later years. It will allow you to function as well as possible as long as possible, through a commonsense approach to nutrition and exercise. The goal of *Thin over 40* is not to "cheat" the aging process. Rather, it is to respectfully acknowledge the aging process and operate within its framework to maximize health and vitality. Notice, I said "healthy and vitality," not "youth." I don't believe it is healthy for someone over forty to be obsessive about "youth." It's not realistic and by doing so you miss out on all of the joys of the age you're in. Each phase of life has its advantages and disadvantages. In our culture, we put far too much attention on the advantages of youth and the disadvantages of age. This relegates those over forty to defeatism and despair. If you spend your forties sad you're no longer thirty, and your fifties sad you're no longer forty, and your sixties sad you're no longer fifty, and on and on, you're living year after year under the weight of sadness. Of course, you could just as easily substitute "angry" or "frustrated" for "sad." The point is, by failing to accept your age and fully live within that age, you miss out on life.

SUCCESS IN ACTION

Today I want you to write down all the positive things about the age you are right now. It doesn't matter what age that is. Having trouble thinking of many? That should give you a clue to how negativism is oppressing your optimism, hope, and joy! Fight back! Accept who you are and where you are in your life.

Now, think ahead to those things you look forward to as you age. Perhaps it is grandchildren or more time to devote to friendships when the hectic pace of life with kids slows down. Perhaps you look forward to travel or a project you've been putting off doing. Look over all the things you desire to do or relationships you wish to pursue. These constitute some of your strongest motivations to maintain your *Thin over 40* lifestyle. You've got a lot of living ahead!

WEEK 12 ❦ DAY 4

Today's Thin Thought: Recognize food as a cheap fix for strained emotions.

Your daily assignments: (*Envision yourself doing each of these today. Smile at how good you'll feel during and after each accomplishment!*)
- I drink lots of water.
- I use my body upon waking.
- I walk for at least forty-five minutes a day.
- I keep track of what I eat and how much.
- I choose healthy fats in moderation.
- I am physically active.
- I eat whole foods.
- I take my vitamins.
- I take my supplements.
- I get a good night's sleep.
- I combat my cravings.
- I cut down on sugar.
- I turn to people, not food.
- I focus on my success.

SETTING THE DAY FOR SUCCESS

Over the past eleven weeks you've been educating yourself on how you used food to feed your emotions and faulty beliefs instead of your body. You've chosen food for comfort, stimulation, reward, relaxation—and occasionally nutrition. These are entrenched behaviors and, as such, are difficult to overcome. Lower your guard and they're bound to reassert themselves. Each of you will need to remain diligent to those situations of emotional eating to which you are particularly vulnerable. You'll need to be proactive in crafting a specific strategy to counter the behavior. Here are a few examples you can use to point the way to your personal solutions:

If you eat as a way to comfort, you don't have to give up the comfort; just give up the food for comfort. Comfort can be found in a variety of ways. Perhaps you can choose an area of the house (instead of the kitchen!) and fashion it for your comfort. Choose a special chair or room of the house. Your goal is to create a comfortable environment, free from food, where you give yourself permission to go when you find yourself in need of comfort. Recognize that you've been using one of your senses—taste—to deal with your need for comfort. There are others. Put on a favorite tape or CD. Light an aromatic candle. Surround the space or the room with objects or pictures that are especially meaningful to you. Invite others into your space whenever appropriate. Don't forget that people and relationships can be your greatest source of comfort!

If you eat for stimulation, you've really chosen a cheap solution because there are so many alternatives out there. Whenever possible, get up and move around for stimulation. Take a walk. Go on an errand. See a friend. These are all ways to combat boredom. Read a good book. Learn a new skill. Complete a task. Engage your mind and your body whenever possible.

If you eat to reward yourself, be honest about this predilection. Why are you feeling you need or deserve a reward? Isn't the action, in and of itself, rewarding enough? Why the need for something more? What are you rewarding yourself for? Getting through the day? Not getting angry at a coworker, your kids, or your spouse? Finding a sale? Your sports team winning? Are those really bona fide reasons to reward yourself? Or do you use the term "reward" as an excuse to eat or to overeat? If you really have something to celebrate, call a friend or share it with a family member. If you want to involve food in the celebration, fine! But plan to enjoy a full meal together and focus on the accomplishment, not on food as a reward for the accomplishment.

If you eat to relax, again, you're in luck. There are so many other ways to wind down. I find this to be one of the most habitual eating behaviors. A person who eats to relax often has no real recognition of the food itself. Instead, it's the act of eating that signals physical or mental relaxation. Some people are so keyed up, they have developed a trigger to signal permission to relax. If that describes you, choose a different trigger. Try using a hobby, something you do with your hands, like putting together models, or a craft, knitting or cross-stitch, as that trigger. You'll still be able to relax and accomplish a worthwhile project! If you have trouble coming up with something suitable, think about tasks or chores you enjoy, where you can go hours without the need to eat. This should point you in a good direction.

SUCCESS IN ACTION

In short, there are other ways to fulfill your need for comfort, stimulation, reward, or relaxation. Instead of castigating yourself for having that need, acknowledge it and determine another way of meeting it besides food. Eventually, you may find that the need diminishes, especially if it was more about the food than the emotional need in the first place. In your journal today, acknowledge which of these reasons is most powerful for you. Write it at the top of your page and then come up with three separate avenues for filling the need that have nothing to do with food.

WEEK 12   🦋   DAY 5

Today's Thin Thought: It's time you lived your own life.

Your daily assignments:
- I drink lots of water.
- I use my body upon waking.
- I walk for at least forty-five minutes a day.
- I keep track of what I eat and how much.
- I choose healthy fats in moderation.
- I am physically active.
- I eat whole foods.
- I take my vitamins.
- I take my supplements.
- I get a good night's sleep.
- I combat my cravings.
- I cut down on sugar.
- I turn to people, not food.
- I focus on my success.

SETTING THE DAY FOR SUCCESS

You may be over forty but most of us have one stubborn little kid still rattling around inside. This "kid" represents some unfilled childhood need. And until we either fill or let go of that need, there he or she stays—never aging, always demanding. Kids like to eat junk food. They're not mature enough to realize that it's bad for them. They want a cookie, not broccoli. They want cake, not tofu. Kids, when they finally slow down long enough to figure out they are hungry, have notoriously little patience until fed. Isn't this the essence of cravings? This pattern was established growing up and it can still dominate today. This is why it's so important that you discern when it's hunger talking or that little kid inside saying, "I want what I want—now!"

It's time to take back control over your eating habits by establishing new ones based upon your maturity and understanding. When your little kid pitches a fit, you can calm him or her by acknowledging that you'll be making adult choices from now on. Those childhood messages no longer have to determine your eating patterns today. From eating everything on your plate to a backlash against brussels sprouts, many of your reactions to food began when you were growing up. Understand that you're no longer growing up—you're grown, and you're able to make positive choices from a position of maturity.

Be prepared for that little kid to perceive your control and maturity as a personal loss. After all, he or she has been setting many of your food rules for years and has become used to being in the driver's seat. As you work through these changes, recognize this could be the source of internal conflict you feel between knowing what you need to do and feeling like doing the exact opposite. You've got to decide who will have the upper hand and control your eating patterns. For continued success in *Thin over 40*, it needs to be you—the adult.

SUCESS IN ACTION

Think back on the significant pattern changes you've made in your eating. What's been the hardest to change? Is there a change you know you should make but seem to be unable to? I'd like you to frame it within the context of you, the adult, and you, the child.

The adult knows what you need to do. The child wants to continue what you've always done. Spend some time today acknowledging that that child exists within you. Can you identify the age? Is there more involved than food? In other words, when you don't eat like your child wants, are other emotions associated with that child? Anger? Rebellion? Sadness? Loss?

Recognize children will often use food to deal with emotions because it's one thing they have under their control. And it is often a way children find to successfully control the adults around them. Watch any young child pitch an absolute fit in the grocery store over some snack item. Then watch the parent give in to the tantrum to avoid further embarrassment. As children gain a sense of their own independence and control, food is often the avenue used to express it. Your own child could be the very thing fighting your best intentions to remain *Thin over 40*. (Childhood issues can be very difficult to work through on your own. If you find yourself unable to assert an adult decision because of past childhood issues, I urge you to seek out a professional counselor or therapist. In many cases, food covers over other issues that can be successfully dealt with through the partnership with a professional. The personal insight gained can positively affect not only your eating habits but your very approach to life. Counseling is what I do because it's what I believe in!)

WEEK 12 ❧ DAY 6

Today's Thin Thought: The way around stress isn't found in a plastic wrapper.

Your daily assignments:
- I drink lots of water.
- I use my body upon waking.

- I walk for at least forty-five minutes a day.
- I keep track of what I eat and how much.
- I choose healthy fats in moderation.
- I am physically active.
- I eat whole foods.
- I take my vitamins.
- I take my supplements.
- I get a good night's sleep.
- I combat my cravings.
- I cut down on sugar.
- I turn to people, not food.
- I focus on my success.

SETTING THE DAY FOR SUCCESS

I cannot emphasize how important it is to develop alternate methods to deal with the stresses in your life. I don't know you. I don't know what you're going through. But I know myself, and I deal with stress daily. A while back, I had so much stress in my life I found myself emotionally and physically fried. Out of that experience, I found my own path to revitalization and health. My recovery took a two-pronged approach. First, I needed to look at how I was living my life and make changes to reduce my stress level. At the time, I was working too many long hours with very little time for myself. I felt so compelled to help others, I forgot that I couldn't give what I didn't have. I forgot that I needed to take time to fill up my own well in order to be available to give to others. Second, I needed to incorporate healthier ways of dealing with the inevitable stress that can't be managed away. Simply put, life happens and must be dealt with. Because of the stress in my life, I was losing my optimism, hope, and joy. I didn't like it when it happened to me, and I don't want it to happen to you.

All through this *Thin over 40* training, you've been looking back over your life and evaluating where you've been, where you are now, and where you want to be. In order to get a handle on stress and mitigate the tremendous emotional and physical damage it does to you, I want you to again take inventory of your life. Identify those areas of activity, relationship, or responsibility that cause you the greatest stress. Then, evaluate honestly whether it is the activity, relationship, or responsibility itself that causes the stress, or the way you've *chosen* to deal with it. When you've made a choice to react with dread, anxiety, frustration, impatience, anger, bitterness, shame, or guilt over something, you can be sure whatever it is will cause you stress. Maybe you are unable to change the thing itself, but you can change how you respond to it.

This may also be a very good time for you to make actual changes in the activity, relationship, or responsibility. For example, you may have taken on a responsibility ten years ago, when circumstances were different, and are still doing it out of a sense of obligation. Consider handing over that responsibility to either another person or the entity that created the responsibility in the first place. Only Supreme Court judges are appointed for life—just because you said "yes" years ago doesn't mean you're committed forever. If it's a source of significant stress in your life, it could be time to accept that and let the responsibility pass to another person.

We've already talked about stressful relationships that may need to change, but what about an activity you're doing? It could be a hobby or fun activity you became involved in because it brought joy and benefit to your life. Now, however, circumstances have changed and you're still doing it out of habit as opposed to enjoyment. Will you believe me when I say, "It shows?" Accept when it is time to move on.

What about a major source of stress—your personal finances? Perhaps over the years you've been adding on to your level of personal debt and the accumulated weight is keeping you up at night. Maybe it's time for you to downsize your house or reevaluate your family budget. There are free consumer counseling services in most major cities that can help you restructure your debt and help you pay off creditors.

Maybe you need to ask others to come onboard and help with some of your existing responsibilities. Maybe you need to look for a different job or change your work shift. We tend to think that the conditions we're in have to stay that way, but often even small changes can make a big difference. I've known people who have made it a goal to leave for work twenty minutes earlier and they arrive twice as early because they've avoided the traffic. Are they getting up earlier? Yes, but twenty minutes isn't really that much, yet the tradeoff in time and stress is enormous. They come in to work less stressed and more optimistic about the day. I've also known people who have moved in order to be closer to work or their children's school. In each case, they looked at what was causing stress and chose specific ways to reduce it, from small changes in time to household moves.

SUCCESS IN ACTION

What's causing stress in your life? List the top three. Now, under each, write "Attitude" and "Action." I'd like you come up with ways you can change your attitude about that stress and ways you can take action to reduce the stress. Think outside the box on this. Be creative in evaluating what you can do to make a positive difference. Ask for feedback from those closest to you, especially those involved in the stress with you, such as family or coworkers. As you encounter that stress, think about that stress being completely gone from your life. How does that feel? Are you sure that's what you want? If it's a relationship, if that person who is causing your stress were out of your life, how would that make you feel? Is there a way to work on the relationship to make it less stressful? Take ownership of your stress and set about implementing those changes that make the most sense in the situation.

WEEK 12   🦋   DAY 7

Today's Thin Thought: You can lead a horse to water, but you can't make it drink.

Your daily assignments:
- I drink lots of water.
- I use my body upon waking.
- I walk for at least forty-five minutes a day.
- I keep track of what I eat and how much.
- I choose healthy fats in moderation.
- I am physically active.
- I eat whole foods.
- I take my vitamins.
- I take my supplements.
- I get a good night's sleep.
- I combat my cravings.
- I cut down on sugar.
- I turn to people, not food.
- I focus on my success.

Weekly Assignment:
- Go grocery shopping for next week.

SETTING THE DAY FOR SUCCESS

Yesterday I asked you to take ownership of your stress. Today I want you to take ownership of your *success*. Over the course of these twelve weeks, I've led you to water, as it were. Only you can decide each day to drink. My heartfelt desire is for you to drink up daily! But only you can make that decision.

You have the tools you need to continue to live a *Thin over 40* life. Those, I can give you. What you must find within yourself is the motivation to implement what you've learned each and every day. In order to help you maintain your commitment and keep your motivation alive, I want you to look over the goals you set for yourself at the beginning of your journey. You may have had health goals or weight goals. You may have wanted to change how you're living so you'll be healthy for your children or grandchildren. You may have decided you're sick and tired of feeling sick and tired all the time. You may have determined that you are going to live the next forty years differently than the first. Whatever the reasons, don't lose sight of those goals.

Also, don't lose sight of the success you've had up to this point. It's all too easy to focus on your failures and lament your mistakes. Don't give in to that kind of thinking! Focusing on failures weighs you down and thwarts your efforts to pick yourself back up. Keep your eyes on the success you've had and allow past successes to pave the way for present and future progress. Acknowledging your successes, will allow you the support to take an honest look at those areas where you desire improvement.

SUCCESS IN ACTION

In your journal today, I want you to rewrite the goals you had for yourself at the beginning of *Thin over 40.* Rewrite them just as they were. Now, look them over and make any changes you'd like, based on what you've learned in the interim. Do you want to modify those goals? Are there some you'd like to add? Are there any that no longer seem as important to you?

Next, write "My Successes" at the top of a page and think back through what you've accomplished. It's perfectly fine to be proud of yourself and what you've done—I am! Record insights, victories, changed habits, new understanding. Then, under your successes, I'd like you to list two areas where you acknowledge additional diligence needs to be applied. By doing this, you are not saying that you are a bad person. On the contrary, you are saying that you are fully confident in your ability to address these issues and find success in them also.

HERO OF THE WEEK

I started out *Thin over 40* by saying that you were my Hero. At the risk of being repetitious, I'd like to say you still are! You've stayed the course for twelve weeks. You've done your assignments and taken a good, hard look at who you are and who you want to be. It hasn't been easy, but you've kept with it. To me, you are a walking definition of courage. Changing parts of yourself so integral to who you are is an act of discovery and bravery. I take strength in your strength and, with that strength, want to encourage you to keep going!

Allow yourself to see yourself as a hero, as this courageous, brave person who has the will and ability to make difficult, personal changes. So many people just don't, and suffer for it. Not you—you've accepted the responsibility for your own health and well-being and are actively pursuing both. Go look yourself in the mirror and say, "You're my hero!"

AFTERWORD

For twelve weeks—eighty-four days—you've been devoting yourself to your goal of *Thin over 40*. Just because this book is ending, your commitment is not! Think of this book as a training course—giving you the tools you need to keep going forward. You've always been the one in charge of your future and your health. It's been my privilege to provide some insight, information, and understanding along the way.

Here are a few things to remember:

- *Keep making baby steps.* You have forty-plus years of habits and patterns to work your way through. Twelve weeks is enough time for you to get solidly on the path, but keep taking those baby steps toward the prize of health and vitality. Remember, this isn't a sprint; you're in it for the long run. And in the long run, you have so much to live *Thin over 40* for!

- *Keep focused on your goals.* This isn't about obsessing every day about food. Being focused means you keep your goals clearly in front of you and allow those goals to motivate the way you live your life, from what you eat to how you feel about yourself.

- *Keep your inner dialogue positive.* When those negative messages start playing in your mind, throw out the tape! You must be your firmest supporter,

your biggest cheerleader, your most consistent
friend. No one else is going to do this but you.

- *Keep making mature choices.* Be the adult. When that
child inside insists upon eating or making choices
you know are not in your best interests, assert
your understanding and maturity by choosing to
live *Thin over 40.* Each mature decision will reinforce the next.

- *Keep believing in yourself.* You have what you need
to achieve success, including the ability to know
when to ask for help on a particular issue. You're
in the driver's seat, but there's no harm in asking
for directions. Know that you are capable of arriv-
ing at and living in your goals.

- *Keep committed to the Five Success Essentials.* For the
last twelve weeks, you've been reading them, recit-
ing them, living them regularly. These should be
well on their way to becoming an essential part of
how you live your life and direct your choices.
Here they are again:

Success Essential #1: Intentional, healthy food
and eating choices
Success Essential #2: Increased physical
movement
Success Essential #3: Nutritional and hormonal
support
Success Essential #4: Restful, curative sleep
Success Essential #5: Proper hydration

As you anchor yourself firmly in these essentials,
you will continue to find success!

Remember also that this book is for you. Review
it. Reread it. Go over a specific week or concept that
still needs fortification. Look over your journal. Expand on your answers. In the back of this book,

you'll find a Resource List. On it are books I've included that might be of further interest to you. If you'd like more information on a specific subject, check out the Resource List and choose one to read next, to continue with your good work.

I so desire for you to integrate these truths in your life, not only for the health of your body but also for your peace of mind. For so many people, weight and food issues have acted as a drag on their optimism, hope, and joy. Live these *Thin over* 40 principles you've been learning these twelve weeks and be free! Unlock yourself from the shackles of your past behavior. You have the keys—now use them!

The focus needs to be on you—on your progress— not on this book. The success lies within *you*. Once this book is on a shelf, what you've learned about yourself, what you've worked on, remains with *you*. You become the walking success story for a *Thin over 40* life.

Please know I'm rooting for you. We're all over forty. We're in this together! I invite you to share your successes and your struggles. You can go online to www.thinover40.com and add your story to others. You can always write to me at The Center for Counseling, PO Box 700, Edmonds, WA 98020.

My very best to you.
Gregory L. Jantz
www.aplaceofhope.com
888-771-5166

RESOURCE LIST

I've included a brief description of several books that you might be interested in pursuing, as part of your continued *Thin over 40* walk. They are listed alphabetically by book title. Look them over and find any that relate specifically to a Key Concept you are especially interested in.

8 Minutes in the Morning: A Simple Way to Lose up to 2 Pounds a Week Guaranteed by Jorge Cruise (New York: HarperResource, 2002). For those of you who want a little more structure to your morning stretching and lifting, this book has excellent exercises with photos. These are interspersed throughout his four-week plan. The information he presents is very much in line with *Thin over 40*.

The 20-Day Rejuvenation Diet Program by Jeffrey Bland, Ph.D. with Sara Benum, M.A. (New York: McGrawHill/Contemporary Books, 1999). This book sets out a specific, twenty-day diet program with preset menus based on whole foods and phytonutrients, which he defines as plant foods and their constituents. It goes over supplements, detoxification, chronic fatigue, candida infections, and oxidant stress. Great for those wanting to undertake a guided program of menus and recipes for each day's meals. (Key Concepts: Food and Mood.)

Adrenal Fatigue: The 21st Century Stress Syndrome by James L. Wilson, N.D., D.C., Ph.D. (Petaluma, Cal.: Smart Publications, 2002). It includes a self-test questionnaire to determine if you have adrenal fatigue and, if so, how severe. Included are plenty of testimonials and detailed physical information. (Key Concept: Adrenal Health.)

The Carbohydrate Addict's Healthy Heart Program: Break Your Carbo-Insulin Connection to Heart Disease by Dr. Richard F. Heller, Dr. Rachael F. Heller, and Dr. Frederic J. Vagnini (New York: Ballantine Books, 2000). This book is specifically for those who experience intense sugar and junk-food cravings—in other words, those who identify themselves as addicted to carbohydrates. While it is written from a fairly technical point of view, it has good information on insulin resistance. (Key Concept: Balance.)

Do You Use Food to Cope? A Comprehensive 15-Week Program for Overcoming Emotional Overeating by Dr. Sheila H. Forman (Writers Club Press, 2002). This book draws on Dr. Forman's experience as a clinical psychologist and eating disorder specialist. It is specific to the concept of emotional eating. (Key Concept: Awareness.)

Eating for Life: Your Guide to Great Health, Fat Loss, and Increased Energy by Bill Phillips (High Print Media, 2003). This new book is featured as part of Bill Phillips's Body for Life series. It looks to be a book full of healthy recipes for all meals, while retaining flavor, texture, and taste.

Fight Fat After Forty: The Revolutionary Three-Pronged Approach That Will Break Your Stress-Fat Cycle and

Make You Healthy, Fit, and Trim for Life by Pamela Peeke, M.D., M.P.H. (New York: Viking Press, 2000). Dr. Peeke identifies toxic stress as a prime factor in excess weight and provides a program for determining your stress profile and eating patterns. She shows you how to become more stress resilient and how to boost your metabolism. (Key Concepts: Adrenal Health and Metabolism.)

Get the Sugar Out: 501 Simple Ways to Cut the Sugar Out of Any Diet by Ann Louise Gittleman (New York: Three Rivers Press, 1996). For those who recognize a need to significantly cut down on the amount of processed sugar in their food choices, this book can help provide inspiration, sugar substitutions, and sugar-free recipes. (Key Concept: Balance.)

Graham Kerr's Creative Choices Cookbook by Graham Kerr (New York: Putnam Publishing Group, 1993). I'll let my friend Graham Kerr speak for himself on why this cookbook is so great: "Individual creativity is the key to having more fun in the kitchen. This book will help you 'reassemble' family favorites by replacing excessive salt, fats, and sugars with lots of aroma, color, and flavor." (Key Concept: Food and Mood.)

Healing the Scars of Emotional Abuse by Gregory L. Jantz (Grand Rapids, MI: Revell, 2003). This is my book that looks at the pervasive yet overlooked problem of emotional abuse. Food is often a chosen method to deal with the accumulated hurts of emotional abuse. This book is a great resource for those wanting to explore the effect of emotional abuse on their own eating patterns and relationship with food.

Is Your Thyroid Making You Fat? The Doctor's 28-Day Diet That Tests Your Metabolism as You Lose Weight by Sanford Siegal, D.O., M.D. (New York, Warner Books, 2001). This book includes important information on hypothyroidism and is a resource for those who suspect a thyroid connection to their weight gain and food choices. The basis for this book is a twenty-eight-day diet that "tests your metabolism as you lose weight." (Key Concept: Metabolism.)

Life is Hard, Food is Easy: The 5-Step Plan to Overcome Emotional Eating and Lose Weight on Any Diet by Linda Spangle, R.N., M.A. (Washington, D.C.: Lifeline Press, 2003). This book is especially suited for those who struggle with emotional eating. The author is the founder of a weight-management program in Denver, Colorado, and she outlines a three-step approach to overcome emotional eating. (Key Concept: Awareness.)

The Metabolic Typing Diet: Customize Your Diet to Your Own Unique Body by William Wolcott and Trish Fahey (New York: Broadway Books, 2002). This book identifies three metabolic types and provides guidelines on specific weight-loss strategies for each. (Key Concept: Metabolism.)

Metabolize: The Personalized Program for Weight Loss by Kenneth Baum with Richard Trubo (New York: Perigee, 2000). This book introduces the idea of metabolic profiles and how to customize your eating to match your profile, with a test included for you to determine what that profile is. (Key Concept: Metabolism.)

Moving Beyond Depression: A Whole-Person Approach to Healing by Gregory L. Jantz with Ann McMurray (Colorado Springs: Shaw Books, 2003). Written from a whole-person perspective, my book takes an honest look at the emotional, environmental, relational, physical, and spiritual causes of depression.

The Nutraceutical Revolution: 20 Cutting-Edge Nutrients to Help You Design Your Own Perfect Whole-Life Program by Richard Firshein, D.O. (New York: Penguin Putnam, 1999). Outlining twenty nutrients to replenish what is missing from our food supply, this book advocates the use of vitamins, minerals, herbs, amino acids, and plant phytochemicals. It defines "nutraceutical" as a nutrient that is applied pharmaceutically. (Key Concept: Adrenal Health.)

Outsmarting the Midlife Fat Cell: Winning Weight Control Strategies for Women by Debra Waterhouse, M.P.H., R.D. (New York: Hyperion, 1999). Sorry guys, this one is specifically for women. It's a gem of a book on the physiological changes that occur as women enter and navigate menopause. (Key Concept: Hormones.)

Prescription for Nutritional Healing: A Practical A-Z Reference to Drug-Free Remedies Using Vitamins, Minerals, Herbs, and Food Supplements, Third Edition by Phyllis A. Balch and James F. Balch, M.D. (New York: Penguin Putnam, 2000). This is a really big book with an A to Z reference guide to vitamins, minerals, herbs, and food supplements. If you want to find out about a supplement, this book is an excellent resource. It's so handy, I don't want to box it into any specific Key Concept!

The Serotonin Solution by Judith J. Wurtman, Ph.D., and Susan Suffes (New York: Ballantine Books, 1996). The premise of this book is that a dip in serotonin levels can cause you to crave carbohydrates. It also goes over emotional eating and specific situation "diets." (Key Concept: Brain Power.)

The Testosterone Syndrome by Eugene Shippen, M.D. and William Fryer (New York: M. Evans and Company, Inc., 1998). The goal of this book is to provide readers with the information they need to reverse male menopause. (Key Concept: Hormones.)

Thyroid Power: 10 Steps to Total Health by Richard L. Shames, M.D., and Karilee Halo Shames, R.N., Ph.D. (New York: HarperResource, 2001) This book includes a questionnaire to help answer whether low thyroid could be responsible for a variety of health symptoms. I recommend it for those who suspect thyroid could be an issue. (Key Concept: Adrenal Health.)

Tired of Being Tired: Rescue, Repair, Rejuvenate by Jesse Lynn Hanley, M.D., and Nancy Deville (New York: Putnam Publishing Group, 2001). Dr. Hanley identifies our high-stress lifestyles as the culprit in adrenal system burnout and presents ten solutions, along with meal plans and recipes. (Key Concept: Adrenal Health.)

The Ultimate Weight Solution: The 7 Keys to Weight Loss Freedom by Dr. Phil McGraw (New York: Free Press, 2003). Dr. Phil is a very popular television psychologist and is the author of other self-help, though non-diet related, books. This book touches a bit on nutrition and exercise, but I found the sections on emotional eating and self-talk to be very helpful. (Key Concept: Awareness.)

The Ultimate Weight Solution Food Guide by Dr. Phil McGraw (New York: Pocket Books, 2003). A companion to his *Ultimate Weight Solution,* This *Food Guide* is absolutely amazing and a tremendous resource. It gives the dietary lowdown on all kinds of foods, including portion size, calories, and grams of protein, carbs, and fats/saturated fats, along with information on cholesterol, sugar, and sodium. It's a treasure trove for those searching for nutritional information on "real food" and name-brand items.

What Fatso Taught Me: Lessons on Weight Loss and Overcoming Overeating by Eric Johnson (Writers Club Press, 2001). The inspirational story of the author's two-hundred-pound weight gain and then loss. It is an honest, revealing book that heralds each person's inner strength and ability to understand personal truth. (Key Concept: Awareness.)

What Your Doctor May Not *Tell You about Menopause: The Breakthrough Book on* Natural *Progesterone* by John R. Lee, M.D. with Virginia Hopkins (New York: Warner Books, 1996). This breakthrough book outlines the benefits of natural progesterone for menopausal and other hormonal symptoms. (Key Concept: Hormones.)

What Your Doctor May Not *Tell You about Premenopause* by John R. Lee, M.D., Jesse Hanley, M.D., and Virginia Hopkins (New York: Warner Books, 1999). A groundbreaking book on the effects of premenopause and hormonal balance from age thirty to fifty. (Key Concept: Hormones.)

SIGNET

Barbara Kraus'

CALORIES AND CARBOHYDRATES

A DICTIONARY LISTING OF OVER 8,500 BRAND NAME AND BASIC FOODS WITH THEIR CALORIE AND CARBOHYDRATE COUNTS

"Complete and comprehensive."
—Gene Shalit

0-451-21384-X

Available wherever books are sold or at
www.penguin.com

S912

Take Control of Your Health Now

THE TRANS FAT REMEDY

THE FIRST CONSUMER GUIDE TO YOUR FAMILY'S BIGGEST HEALTH THREAT

by Deborah Mitchell

Uncover the health risks that the labels don't reveal to get the truth about trans fats—where to find them and how to avoid them.

IDENTIFY WHICH FOODS CONTAIN TRANS FATS

•

LEARN WAYS TO SIGNIFICANTLY REDUCE
TRANS FATS IN YOUR DIET

•

GET DETAILED GUIDELINES AND STRATEGIES FOR FINDING
DELICIOUS, NUTRITIOUS ALTERNATIVES TO TRANS FAT-RICH
FOODS IN SUPERMARKETS AND RESTAURANTS

•

PROTECT YOUR FAMILY BY LEARNING TRANS FAT-FREE
RECIPES AND MENUS FOR HEALTHY MEALS

0-451-21272-X

**Available wherever books are sold or at
www.penguin.com**